Articulation and Phonological Disorders

A Book of Exercises

Second Edition

Ken M. Bleile

Articulation and Phonological Disorders

A Book of Exercises

Second Edition

Ken M. Bleile

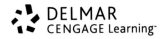

DELMAR
CENGAGE Learning·

Australia • Brazil • Japan • Korea • Mexico • Singapore • Spain • United Kingdom • United States

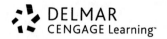

**Articulation and Phonological Disorders:
A Book of Exercises, Second Edition**
Ken M. Bleile

For product information and technology assistance, contact us at
Cengage Learning Customer & Sales Support, 1-800-354-9706

For permission to use material from this text or product,
submit all requests online at **www.cengage.com/permissions**
Further permissions questions can be emailed to
permissionrequest@cengage.com

ISBN-13: 978-1-56593-688-1

ISBN-10: 1-56593-688-4

Delmar
Executive Woods
5 Maxwell Drive
Clifton Park, NY 12065
USA

Cengage Learning is a leading provider of customized learning solutions with office locations around the globe, including Singapore, the United Kingdom, Australia, Mexico, Brazil, and Japan. Locate your local office at **international.cengage.com/region**

Cengage Learning products are represented in Canada by Nelson Education, Ltd.

To learn more about Delmar, visit **www.cengage.com/delmar**

Purchase any of our products at your local college store or at our preferred online store **www.ichapters.com**

Notice to the Reader

Printed in the United States of America
7 8 9 10 11   16 15 14 13 12

CONTENTS

Preface to the Second Edition

Disorders of articulation and phonology affect persons of all ages and cultures. An individual with an articulation and phonological disorder may be an infant with a severe medical disorder who fails to babble, a previously tracheostomized toddler who speaks her first word near her second birthday, a preschooler whose expressive vocabulary consists of 10 words, a speaker of an African-American dialect who also experiences speech difficulties, a bright school-aged child who stumbles over longer scientific words, or an adult who lisps when he becomes tired or nervous. The speech outcomes of persons with articulation and phonological disorders are varied. Those with milder forms of the disorder may improve spontaneously or with only small amounts of treatment, with those at the other end of the severity spectrum possibly never acquiring speech as a primary means of communication.

This workbook is concerned with articulation and phonological development and its disorders. Exercises offer opportunities to study both typical development, as well as the speech of persons with mild to severe disorders. Only the vocalizations of clients not yet using words for communication are excluded from consideration because of the difficulty in using phonetic transcription to represent their sound making.

The workbook is practical in nature and eclectic in spirit. Either the entire book or individual chapters may be used as modules in clinical settings, as the problem-based learning component in classes on articulation and phonological disorders, for self-study, and as part of linguistic and psychology courses on child development. The book's conceptual and theoretical underpinnings are sufficiently broad that it can be used in conjunction with any number of different textbooks and by persons from a wide variety of theoretical backgrounds. The problems and questions in each exercise provide possible directions for study. However, readers who so desire may use the speech samples for their own purposes.

Readers familiar with the first edition of this workbook will notice many changes. The present edition includes more than double the original number of exercises, has longer speech samples, considers speech from a wider range of persons, and places greater emphasis on treatment principles and therapeutic activities. The entire text has been completely rewritten to follow the format of *The Manual of Articulation and Phonological Disorders* (Bleile, 1995). Text from the manual is used here as chapter introductions, which allows persons reading both the manual and the workbook to perform the exercises without having to continually switch between the two books. The inclusion of text from the manual also makes the workbook more useful for persons pursuing independent study and those wishing to perform the workbook exercises in conjunction with another textbook.

The workbook is organized into five sections. The first section focuses on basic conceptual and terminological issues, including distinctive features, speech sounds, suprasegmentals, and modification of symbols. The second section considers common characteristics and individual differences in typical development. Exercises in this section provide opportunities to analyze phonetic inventories, error patterns, consonants and consonant clusters, dialect and second language, and acquisition strategies.

The remaining three sections focus on assessment, treatment principles, and facilitative techniques. Chapters in the third section contain assessment exercises on measures of severity and intelligibility, developmental age norms, better abilities, and related analysis. The chapters in the fourth section consider treatment principles involved in the selection of goals, treatment targets, administrative decisions, and methods to assess treatment progress. The chapters in the fifth section describe such facilitative techniques as bombardment, increasing awareness, facilitating syllables and words, and indirect and direct techniques. The workbook concludes with references, an appendix containing answers to the exercises, two appendixes containing longer speech samples, and an appendix describing transcription conventions.

Acknowledgments

It is a pleasure to acknowledge those who assisted in the development of this book. My special thanks is to the persons whose speech serves as the basis for the exercises. My hope is that they feel that some good has come from their experiences. I also wish to thank Palmer Curtis and Bruce Tomblin for encouraging my early interest in child phonology and John Bernthal for encouraging me to submit the first edition of this workbook to Singular Publishing Group. I extend my deep thanks to Brian Goldstein and Patricia Dukes for coauthoring chapters, and to Katherine Carpenter, Karla Izuka, Jihee Kim, Robin Seo, and Mary Wolfe for providing speech samples for exercises. My thanks also go to the students in articulation and phonology courses at the University of Hawaii for their insightful comments and suggestions, especially Maggie Reyes, the best of student editors. Lastly, as always, I wish to thank Terry and Judy for making home the place I'd rather be.

For Terry

SECTION
I

Basic Concepts and Terminology

OVERVIEW

Transcription is an important (if somewhat boring) topic in the care for persons with articulation and phonological disorders. Inaccurate transcription of a client's speech can result in mistaken diagnoses and misdirected treatment plans, which waste both the client's and clinician's time. The chapters in this section contain exercises on concepts and terminology that arise during the transcription of the speech of persons with articulation and phonological disorders. Individual chapters contain exercises on distinctive features, speech sounds, suprasegmentals, and modification of symbols. The assumption in the discussion that follows is that readers are familiar with much of the material, so that the presentation is more a review than an introduction to new ideas.

Articulation and Phonological Disorders

Not all speech problems are articulation and phonological disorders. The types of speech problems addressed in this book meet four criteria:

1. The speech is not directly attributable to physical damage to the speech mechanism, sensory systems, peripheral nervous system, or central nervous system.

2. The speech is similar to that of children without articulation and phonological disorders.

3. The speech is not the result of dialect.

4. The speech is considered disordered either by the client and/or members of the client's community.

CHAPTER
1

Distinctive Features

Distinctive features provide an important means of organizing sounds into sound classes. Although there are a number of distinctive feature approaches from which clinicians can choose, by far the oldest and most influential is that depicted in the familiar consonant and vowel charts shown in Tables 1–1 and 1–2, respectively (International Clinical Phonetics and Linguistics Association, 1992a). For example, according to these charts [b] has the features of voice, bilabial, and stop. Similarly, [i] has the features of close, front, and spread. Although the distinctive feature systems shown in Tables 1–1 and 1–2 are well suited to most clinical situations, the exercises in the book do not depend crucially on their use. Other feature systems the reader might want to explore appear in Chomsky and Halle (1968), Ladefoged (1983), Stevens and Keyser (1989), and Stoel-Gammon and Dunn (1985).

Lastly, there are several additional distinctive features not shown in Tables 1–1 and 1–2 that offer clinically useful ways to classify sounds. These classes are defined below.

Approximant	Glides and liquids
Labial	Bilabial and labiodental consonants
Obstruent	Oral stops, fricatives, and affricates
Sibilant	Alveolar and postalveolar fricatives and affricates
Sonorant	Nasals, liquids, and glides
Strident	Labiodental, alveolar, and post-alveolar fricatives and affricates
Diphthong	Sequence of vowels in which only one is syllabic (in this book the term *vowel* is generally used to indicate both diphthongs and pure vowels)

TABLE 1–1. Consonants of American English.

Manner of Production	Place of Production							
	Bilabial	Labiodental	Interdental	Alveolar	Postalveolar	Palatal	Velar	Glottal
Stop								
Oral	p b			t d			k g	
Nasal	m			n			ŋ	
Fricative		f v	θ ð	s z	ʃ ʒ			h
Affricate					tʃ dʒ			
Liquid								
Central				r				
Lateral				l				
Glide	w					j		

TABLE 1–2. Vowels of American English.

Height	Place			
	Front +Sprd	Central	− Rnd	Back + Rnd
Close	i			u
Close mid	ɪ eɪ		ʊ	oʊ
Open mid	ɛ æ	ə	ʌ	ɔ
Open	a			ɑ

Additional Comments:

1. +Sprd = lips spread, − Rnd = lips unrounded, + Rnd = lips rounded

2. The close spread and rounded vowels (which are often pronounced as diph-thongs) are transcribed as [i] and [u].

3. Additional diphthongs: [ɔɪ] = tongue begins as for [ɔ] and moves toward [i], [aɪ] = tongue begins as for [a] and moves toward [i], [aʊ] = tongue be-gins as for [a] and moves toward [ʊ], [ɚ] = tongue shape has both [ə]-like and [r]-like qualities

Exercise 1–1: Distinctive Features

Clinical care often proceeds more quickly if the clinician is aware of the classes to which sounds belong. For example, a client might have difficulty producing the first sounds in *pie*, *top*, and *key*. If the clinician fails to realize that these three different sounds all belong to a single sound class (voiceless stops), he or she might think that the client has three speech problems and might, based on this analysis, be forced to develop three remediation plans. However, a more knowledgeable clinician understands that what the client likely needs is a single remediation plan designed to treat one class of sounds. This and the following exercise provide practice using distinctive features to classify speech sounds. The first exercise asks you to identify speech sounds within particular sound classes, and the next exercise asks you to identify sound classes based on the sounds they contain.

Consonant and Vowel Charts

Consonant and vowel charts give articulatory definitions of speech sounds. For example, [t] is defined as alveolar, voiceless, and stop. However, articulatory definitions should be considered with caution, as a sound perceived as [t] can actually be produced in a variety of ways. For example, [t] can be made with the tongue tip behind either the two upper front teeth or the two lower front teeth.

QUESTIONS

1. Which sound classes are obstruents? *This is an example and is answered for you.*

2. Which consonant places of production are labial?

3. Which vowels are front?

4. Which consonant is a voiceless alveolar fricative?

5. Which feature distinguishes [f] from [v]?

6. Which features distinguish [p] from [d]?

7. Which feature distinguishes [i] from [eɪ]?

8. Which sound is voiced, interdental, and fricative?

9. Which sound is back, unrounded, and open mid?

10. Which sound is palatal?

11. Which sound is liquid and central?

12. Which sounds are voiceless stops?

13. Which vowel is close and spread?

14. Which sounds are approximants?

15. Which sound is lateral?

Answer Sheet for Exercise 1–1: Distinctive Features

1. **obstruents:** oral stops, fricatives, affricates

2. **labial:**

3. **front:**

4. **voiceless alveolar fricative:**

5. **[f] from [v]:**

6. **[p] from [d]:**

7. **[i] from [eɪ]:**

8. **voiced, interdental, fricative:**

9. **back, unrounded, and open mid:**

10. **palatal:**

11. **liquid and central:**

12. **voiceless stops:**

13. **close and spread:**

14. **approximants:**

15. **lateral:**

Exercise 1–2: Distinctive Features

An understanding of a client's speech abilities often requires identifying the sound class to which particular groups of sounds belong. This exercise provides you practice in this important aspect of clinical care.

One From Another

Unless specifically asked, it isn't necessary to list all of a sound's distinctive features. To illustrate, the complete list of distinctive features for [l] is voiced, alveolar, liquid, and lateral. However, as [l] is the only lateral in English, the distinctive feature lateral is sufficient to distinguish [l] from all other sounds.

PROBLEM

Use distinctive features to define the sounds and groups of sounds listed on the answer sheet. *The first word is an example and is answered for you.*

Answer Sheet for Exercise 1–2: Distinctive Features

1. **eɪ:** front, close mid, spread

2. **l:**

3. **p t k:**

4. **u:**

5. **l r:**

6. **ə:**

7. **i:**

8. **eɪ ɛ:**

9. **l r j w:**

10. **æ:**

11. **k g ŋ :**

12. **s t ʃ :**

13. θ **ð:**

14. **t d s z n l r:**

15. **w j:**

CHAPTER
2

Speech Sounds

Speech sounds (consonants, vowels, and diphthongs) are often the major focus of evaluation and treatment. The sounds of American English were presented in Tables 1–1 and 1–2. A transcription that includes only the sounds in Tables 1–1 and 1–2 is called a **broad transcription**. A more detailed transcription of speech is called a **narrow transcription**. The exercises in this chapter require broad transcription, while those in Chapter 4 provide practice with the special symbols and diacritics used in narrow transcription.

Exercise 2–1: Speech Sounds

The problems in this section provide opportunities to brush up rusty transcription skills. Transcribe the words using only the sounds included in Tables 1–1 and 1–2.

Minor Differences

You'll likely encounter many instances in this book where your transcription differs in minor ways from that shown in a speech sample or answer sheet. For example, you might transcribe *hanger* with a [g], and the answer sheet may not contain that sound. Or you might transcribe the vowel in *May* as [e] and the speech sample may show it to be a diphthong. When such discrepancies arise, ask yourself if they are clinically relevant. Many small differences exist in how people transcribe speech. The vast majority are attributable to dialect, individual variations in speech, and transcriber error. Most of these minor differences have little or no clinical relevance.

PROBLEM

Transcribe each of the words on the answer sheet as you would say them carefully in isolation or, better yet, have someone say them carefully and slowly, and you transcribe that person's speech. *The first word is an example and is transcribed for you.*

Answer Sheet for Exercise 2–1: Speech Sounds

1. **cat:** kæt

2. **thin:**

3. **unite:**

4. **brew:**

5. **giving:**

6. **fingernail polish:**

7. **century:**

8. **please:**

9. **winter:**

10. **between:**

Exercise 2–2: Speech Sounds

After completing the previous exercise, compare your transcription to that provided in the back of the book, circling the sounds you mistranscribed. If you need additional practice, transcribe the following words, giving special attention to the sounds you transcribed in error.

PROBLEM

As in the previous exercise, transcribe each word as you would say it carefully in isolation or, better yet, have someone say the words carefully and slowly, and you transcribe that person's speech.

Answer Sheet for Exercise 2–2: Speech Sounds

1. **dog:**

2. **money:**

3. **sat:**

4. **judge:**

5. **mastering:**

6. **phonetic symbols:**

7. **sheep:**

8. **loud:**

9. **ketchup:**

10. **yes:**

CHAPTER
3

Suprasegmentals

Suprasegmentals are aspects of speech larger than the speech sound (segment). The suprasegmentals considered in this chapter are assimilation, syllables, and stress.

Why Articulation and Phonological Disorders?

Articulation disorders result from problems in speech motor control, while phonological disorders result from problems in language knowledge. Research does not yet provide a means to reliably distinguish on a daily clinical basis be-tween articulation and phonological sources of speech problems. In this book, problems in speech are called **articulation and phonological disorders** so as not to bias the discussion toward either a speech motor or language perspective.

ASSIMILATION

The influence of one sound on another is called **assimilation**. **Progressive assimilation** is the influence of an earlier occurring sound on a later occurring one, as when [r] is pronounced with rounded lips in *shriek* due to the presence of lip rounding of [ʃ]. **Regressive assimilation** is the influence of a later occurring sound on an earlier occurring one, as when [n] is pronounced as a dental consonant in *tenth* due to the presence of [θ].

SYLLABLES

Syllable structure is the organization of syllables. To illustrate, the following is a possible depiction of the syllable structure of *between*:

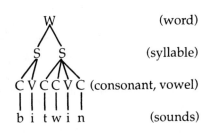

W   (word)

S   S   (syllable)

C V C C V C (consonant, vowel)

b i t w i n (sounds)

15

As syllables are always part of words, many times the word level is not included in the depiction of syllable structure. Other levels may be added or deleted depending on the purpose of the analysis. For example, if needed, a level of distinctive features might be added below that of sounds. Alternately, if the purpose is to describe **syllable sequences** within words and phrases, only the consonant and vowel level is described, and a period (.) is used to indicate syllable boundaries. To illustrate, the syllable sequence of *between* is CV.CCVC.

STRESS

Stress is "the beat" of words and phrases. For example, primary stress in *balloon* occurs on the second syllable. Primary stress is indicated by placing a line above the vowel in the appropriate syllable; syllables receiving lesser stress are left unmarked. To illustrate, stress in *balloon* is *ballóon*.

Exercise 3–1: Suprasegmentals

A client's success (or failure) in making a sound often is influenced by the presence of other sounds in a word or phrase. A client, for example, may pronounce [k] in *king* but not in *key*, because the pronunciation of [k] is facilitated by the presence of [ŋ], as both are made at the same place of production.

On the other hand, the same client might be unable to produce [t] in words such as *take*, because the presence of [k] causes the client to pronounce [t] as [k]. In this exercise you are asked to identify types of assimilations and to use your knowledge of phonetics to help explain why such assimilations occur.

QUESTIONS

1. What is progressive assimilation? *This is an example and is answered for you.*

2. What is regressive assimilation?

3. Why is [n] usually a dental consonant in the word *tenth*? (**Hint:** This question and the next three questions are asking you both to identify the type of assimilation—progressive or regressive—and to provide a reasonable phonetic explanation for why the assimilation occurs.)

4. Why is [r] usually voiceless in the word *pride*?

5. Explain in your own words why some speakers say *sandwich* as *samwich*.

6. Explain in your own words why *something* is often pronounced with a [p] between [m] and [θ]. (**Hint:** The same explanation illustrates why most speakers place a [p] between [m] and [s] in *Chomsky*, leading that well-known linguist's name to be pronounced *Chompsky*.)

7. Explain in your own words why some children pronounce the final [d] in *bead* as [b].

8. Explain in your own words why a child might pronounce *peak* as [kik].

9. *For discussion:* Explain in your own words why a child might correctly pronounce [t] as [t] when the sound occurs before front vowels (for example, in words such as *tea*), but might pronounce [t] as [k] when the sound occurs before back vowels (for example, in words such as *two*).

Answer Sheet for Exercise 3–1: Suprasegmentals

1. **progressive assimilation:** influence of an earlier sound on a later sound

2. **regressive assimilation:** influence of a later occuring sound on an earlier one.

3. **tenth:** the presence of /θ/ makes /n/ a dental consonant

4. **pride:** progressive assimilation; the /p/'s voicing makes the /r/ voiceless

5. **sandwich:**

6. **something:** progressive assimilation; /m/ is produced bilabially & so is /p/, the only difference is /p/ is released & the /θ/ forces the lips to open & can sometimes release air sounding like a /p/.

7. **bead:**

8. **peak:** regressive assimilation; anticipation of the final /k/ makes the child produce the /p/ as /k/.

9. *For discussion:* /t/ is an interdental sound produced at the front of the mouth. So when paired with a back vowel like /u/ sometimes a back consonant will result like /k/

Exercise 3–2: Suprasegmentals

Syllables play an important role in the assessment and treatment of articulation and phonological disorders. Many clients in earlier stages of development, for example, have difficulty pronouncing voiceless sounds in the beginning of syllables and words, leading them to say words such as *pea* and *toe* as *bee* and *doe*, respectively. Many clients also have difficulty pronouncing voiced sounds at the end of syllables, which leads them to pronounce words such as *pig* and *bib* as *pick* and *bip*, respectively. Other influences of syllables on speech can be found at similar and more advanced stages in development. This exercise deals with syllable structure and the following exercise covers syllable sequences.

PROBLEM

Transcribe the first six words on the answer sheet and describe their syllable structure, placing S (for syllable) above your phonetic transcription and drawing lines between the speech sounds and the appropriate S. *The first word is an example and is transcribed for you.* (**Hint:** Describe the syllable structures of the words as they are pronounced slowly and carefully.)

Next, describe the syllable structure of the phrases *it is* and *this time* when spoken slowly and carefully. Then indicate how those structures change when the phrases are spoken more quickly and casually. (**Hint:** Say the phrases several times quickly, listening carefully to the last consonant in *it* and *this*.)

For discussion: First, consider how syllable structure changed in the phrases *it is* and *this time*. Next, describe in your own words how you might use syllable structure to facilitate acquisition of [st] in the speech of client who is able to pronounce word initial [t] and word final [s].

Answer Sheet for Exercise 3–2: Suprasegmentals

1. **diaper:** S S

daɪ pɚ

2. **pretend:**

3. **banana:**

4. **branches:**

5. **abalone:**

6. **winter:**

7. **it is:**

8. **this time:**

9. *For discussion:*

Exercise 3–3: Suprasegmentals

Not all sequences of sounds in syllables are equally easy or difficult. For example, all other matters being equal, a client is likely to have less difficulty with a CV sequence (as in *two*) than a CCCVC sequence (as in *strap*). This exercise provides opportunities to identify sequences of syllables in words.

PROBLEM

Describe the words on the answer sheet in terms of the sequence of consonants and vowels within the syllables. Indicate syllable boundaries with a period (.). *The first word is an example and is described for you.* (**Hint:** Indicate syllable boundaries as you would say the words and phrase slowly and carefully).

Answer Sheet for Exercise 3–3: Suprasegmentals

1. **below:** CV.CV

2. **Sunday:**

3. **infatuate:**

4. **eye:**

5. **winter:**

6. **egg:**

7. **etch:**

8. **powerful emotions:**

9. **spread:**

10. **knight:**

<hr>

Exercise 3–4: Suprasegmentals

Stress is yet another dimension of speech that can influence a client's ability to pronounce words and phrases. For example, because English is a language that favors words with stress on the first syllable (called a **trochaic stress pattern**), clients in earlier stages in development may delete the first unstressed syllable in words such as *banana* and *beginning*, and more advanced clients may continue to have difficulty with unstressed syllables in longer words such as *refrigerator* and *astronomy*. This exercise provides opportunities to learn to identify primary stress in multisyllabic words.

PROBLEM

Identify which syllable in each word receives primary stress. Although it is not necessary to do so, you may also wish to capitalize all the letters in the syllable that receives primary stress. *The first word is an example and is described for you.* (**Hint:** If you have problems identifying the syllable that receives primary stress, say each word aloud several times, changing the syllable that receives primary stress. For example, pronounce *balloon* with exaggerated primary stress as *BA lloon* and *ba LLOON*. The pronunciation that sounds most natural is likely the one with primary stress in the correct syllable.)

<hr>

Answer Sheet for Exercise 3–4: Suprasegmentals

1. **begin:** be GIN

2. **bishop:**

3. **happiness:**

4. **astronomy:**

5. **telescope:**

6. **meadow:**

7. **failure:**

8. **apologize:**

9. **believer:**

10. **astrophysics:**

CHAPTER
4

Modification of Symbols

Sometimes clinicians need more phonetic details about a person's speech than is provided by the symbols listed in Tables 1–1 and 1–2. A set of special symbols and diacritics have been developed to help transcribe the speech of persons with articulation and phonological disorders (**special symbols** are non-English sounds and **diacritics** are modifications made to English sounds). A complete set of special symbols and diacritics is provided in the appendix of this chapter. Those that are used most commonly in clinical care are listed in Table 4–1.

Special notations are another useful adjunct to clinical care. Extensive use of special notations is rare in clinical practice. Some notations are necessary, however, and others, although not necessary, are extremely convenient. The most commonly encountered notations are described next.

[ ] and / /

Square brackets indicate a phonetic transcription, and slashes indicate a phonemic transcription. Single sounds, groups of sounds, and entire words or phrases can be placed within brackets or slashes. Square brackets imply nothing about the phonological status of the sounds being transcribed, whereas slashes (e.g., *bee* as /bi/) indicate that the sounds being transcribed are phonemes—that is, the sounds distinguish one

word from another in the client's speech, just as "p" and "b" do in adult English *pea* and *bee*. Determining which sounds are phonemes in a client's speech is a controversial procedure that is seldom performed in most clinical settings. For this reason, unless a phonemic analysis of the client's speech has been performed, it usually is better to enclose a transcription in square brackets rather than in slashes.

x → y and y/x

The literal meaning of the first notation is "x becomes y," and the literal meaning of the second notation is "y for x." Both types of notations provide simple ways to describe speech changes. For example, the pronunciation of [d] for [t] is indicated as d/t using an x/y notation. The arrow notation is used most often in linguistically oriented approaches, and the slash notation is used in more traditional approaches.

x → y/z

This algebraic-looking notation literally means "x becomes y in the environment of z." The notation is used to describe how a phonetic or word environment affects production of speech. The "x" and "y" can be any articulation and phonological unit—features, consonants, vowels, individual sounds, syllables, or stress.

TABLE 4–1. Commonly special symbols and diacritics.

Symbols	Definitions	Examples
[ɸ] [β]	* Bilabial fricatives (two lips approximate each other)	ɸ β
[̪]	Labiodental oral and nasal stops (upper teeth to lower lip)	p̪ b̪ m̪
[̪]	Interdentalized (also called lisped) (tongue tip/blade between teeth)	t̪ l̪
[ʔ]	Glottal stop (stop produced at vocal folds)	ʔ
[°]	Unaspirated (normally aspirated voiceless stops produced without aspiration)	p°
[̭]	Bladed (produced with tongue blade)	s̭ z̭
[ɹ]	[w]-coloring ([r] with a [w]-like quality)	r
[ls]	Lateralized [s] and [z], respectively (air over the sides of tongue)	ls lz

* = Whenever two symbols are presented, the first is unvoiced and the second is voiced.

A Quick Summary

Here is a quick summary of how information contained in the first four chapters is used throughout the book:

- Exercise questions about **distinctive features** ask you to describe sounds in terms of their distinctive features (example: [b] is a voiced, bilabial, oral stop)
- Exercise questions about **speech sounds** ask you to describe speech in terms of the sounds it contains (example: *meat* and *moo* both contain [m] in word initial position)
- Exercise questions about **assimilation** ask you to describe the effect of one sound on another (example: [r] is usually voiceless in *pride* because it follows voiceless [p])
- Exercise questions about **syllable structure** ask you to describe speech in terms of the organization within syllables (example: the syllable structure of *bee* is:

- Exercise questions about **syllable sequences** ask you to describe words in terms of consonants and vowels (example: the syllable sequence of *banana* is CV.CV.CV and the syllable sequence of *bug* is CVC)
- Exercise questions about **stress** ask you to describe words in terms of their stress patterns (example: primary stress in *money* occurs on the first syllable (*MOney*)
- The few exercise questions about **special symbols and diacritics** ask you to identify symbols and diacritics used in the transcription of speech (for example, [x] is a voiceless velar fricative that sometimes replaces [k])
- The few exercise questions on **special notations** ask you to use a simple notation to describe some aspect of speech (for example, a traditional notation of [w] for [r] is w/r)

The "z" typically is a distinctive feature, consonant, vowel, a **syllable boundary** (symbolized as "S"), or a **word boundary** (symbolized as "#"). For example, within this notation the pronunciation of liquids as glides word initially would be indicated as follows:

liquids → glides/#__

~

The squiggly line (called a tilde) indicates an alternation in pronunciation. It is a handy shorthand way to describe the speech of clients who vary in how they say given sounds and syllables. For example, a client might pronounce *pea* as [pi] and [bi], in which case the alternation between [p] and [b] would be indicated as pi~bi or [pi~bi]. Although it is possible to use this notation to describe alternations in distinctive features, stress patterns, and word shapes, the tilde is more commonly used to describe alternations affecting sounds and, less often, syllables.

Exercise 4–1: Modification of Symbols

This exercise provides practice in identifying special symbols and diacritics commonly encountered in clinical care.

QUESTIONS

1. What is the symbol for lateralized [s]? *This is an example and is answered for you.*
2. What is the symbol for labiodental [m]?
3. What is the symbol for glottal stop?
4. What is the symbol for unaspirated [t]?
5. What is the symbol for bladed [z]?
6. Define [β].
7. Define [x].
8. Define [↑].
9. Define [ɾ].
10. Define [fŋ].

Answer Sheet for Exercise 4–1: Modification of Symbols

1. **lateralized [s]:** [ǁs]

2. **labiodental [m]:**

3. **glottal stop:**

4. **unaspirated [t]:**

5. **bladed [z]:**

6. **[β]:**

7. **[x]:**

8. **[↑]:**

9. **[ɾ]:**

10. **[fŋ]:**

Exercise 4–2: Modification of Symbols

Special notations are a convenient type of shorthand. This exercise provides practice in their use.

QUESTIONS

1. Make a phonemic transcription of "k" in *key*. *This is an example and is answered for you.*
2. Make a phonetic transcription of "k" in *key*.
3. Make a phonetic transcription of bilabial oral stops.
4. Make a phonetic transcription of the word *duke*.
5. Indicate using both linguistically based and traditional notations that a client says [t] as [d].
6. Indicate using both linguistically based and traditional notations that a client says liquids as glides.
7. Indicate using both linguistically based and traditional notations that a client deletes the second consonant in clusters containing two consonants.

8. Indicate that a client says [g] as [k] at the ends of words.

9. Indicate that a client says voiceless fricatives as voiced fricatives between vowels.

10. Indicate that a client says two as [tu] or [du].

Answer Sheet for Exercise 4–2: Modification of Symbols

1. **phonemic:** /k/

2. **phonetic:** [k]

3. **bilabial oral stops:** [p][b]

4. *duke:* [duk]   ✓

5. **[t] as [d]:** t →d   or t/d

6. **liquids as glides:** liquids →glides   or   liquids/glides

7. **deletion:** CC→CD   CD/CC

8. **[g] as [k]:** g→k/___#

9. **between vowels:** voiceless fricatives → voiced/V___V

10. **[tu] or [du]:** two is pronounced tu~du

APPENDIX

Non-English Symbols and Diacritics

A. Place of Production

[ɸ] [β]	* Bilabial fricatives (two lips approximate each other)	ɸ β
[ˏ]	Labiodental oral and nasal stops (upper teeth to lower lip)	p̪ b̪ m̪
[̄]	Dentolabial plosives and nasal (lower teeth to upper lip)	p̄ b̄ m̄
[ˌ]	Interdentalized (also called lisped) (tongue tip/blade between teeth)	t̪ l̪
[̮]	Bidental (teeth approximated)	h̬ u̬
[̰]	Bidental percussive (teeth brought percussively together)	t̬ d̬
[ɲ]	Palatal nasal (nasal stop made at palatal region)	ɲ
[x] [ɣ]	Velar fricatives (fricatives produced in the velar region)	x ɣ
[fŋ]	Velopharyngeal fricative (fricative made in velopharyngeal region)	fŋ
[ʔ]	Glottal stop (stop produced at vocal folds)	ʔ

B. Manner of Production

[↔]	Labial spreading (lips spread)	s̤↔ d̤↔
[ˌ]	Unrounded (lips at rest, unpursed)	w̲
[ˣ]	Denasal (little air through nose)	n̆
[ˣ]	Nasal escape (air through nose)	p̆ d̆
[ˌ]	Bladed (produced with tongue blade)	s̬ z̬
[r̯]	[w]-coloring ([r] with a [w]-like quality)	r̯
[ɾ]	Flap (quick stop-like consonant as in "butter")	ɾ

[ǀs]	Lateralized [s] and [z], respectively (air over the sides of tongue)	ǀs ǀz
[̎]	Stronger production (produced with greater force than is typical)	f̎
[m̜]	Weaker production (produced with less force than is typical)	m̜
[↑]	Whistled (high pitched sound)	s̑↑
[t̤]	Wet sound (produced with excess saliva)	t̤

C. Airstream

| [↓] | Ingressive (air moves inward) | p↓ |
| [(X)] | Silent or "mouthing" (no sound produced) | (s) |

D. Vocal Fold Activity

[̗] [̗]	Pre and postvoicing of sounds (voicing begins or ends later than expected)	z̗
[₍ ₎]	Partial devoicing (normally voiced sound is partially devoiced)	z₍ₒ₎
[₍ ₎]	Partial voicing (normally voiceless sound is partially voiced)	f₍ᵥ₎
[ʰ]	Preaspiration (sound begins with aspiration)	ʰp
[°]	Unaspirated (normally aspirated voiceless stops produced without aspiration)	p̊

E. Syllables and Stress

[ˌ]	Syllabic (consonant standing as a syllable)	l̩
[.]	Syllable boundary (separation between syllables)	bi.twin
[´]	Primary stress (syllable with main stress)	bitwín

Compiled from "Recommended Phonetic Symbols: Extensions of the IPA," by the International Clinical Phonetics and Linguistics Association, 1992b, *Clinical Linguistics and Phonetics, 6*, 259–261.

* = Whenever two symbols are presented, the first is unvoiced and the second is voiced.

SECTION
II

Typical Development: Common Characteristics and Individual Differences

OVERVIEW

The care of persons with articulation and phonological disorders begins with the study of typical articulation and phonological development. **Typical development** serves as a metric against which to evaluate the speech of persons with possible articulation and phonological disorders. For most clinicians, typical development also is an important source of treatment principles and facilitative techniques.

Although many different analyses of articulation and phonological development are possible, the three most directly relevant to clinical care are the analysis of phonetic inventories, error patterns, and acquisition of consonants and consonant clusters. Additionally, identification of typical dialect and second language patterns is necessary to distinguish disorder from language differences, and the analysis of acquisition strategies, although not performed in many clinical settings, is important because of the insight it provides into cognitive mechanisms that underlie articulation and phonological development.

The acquisition of articulation and phonology occurs over a period of many years. For clinical purposes, in this book this long period is divided into the four broad stages described below and summarized in Table II–1.

Stage 1

This stage occurs in typically developing infants from birth to approximately 12 months of age. During this stage vocalizations are seldom, if ever, used for referential purposes. Activities such as cooing and babbling allow the child to "practice the vocal mechanism." Articulation and phonological care of clients in this developmental stage focuses primarily on facilitating the acquisition of vocal skills that underlie later speech development. Because Stage 1 vocalizations do not lend themselves well to transcription using standard phonetic symbols, this stage is not discussed in this book.

TABLE II–1. Primary characteristics of four stages in articulation and phonological development.

Stages	Age Range in Typically Developing Children	Primary Characteristics
Stage 1	0–12 ms	Vocalizations seldom if ever used for referential purposes
Stage 2	12–24 ms	Small expressive vocabulary (less than 100 words)
Stage 3	2–5 yrs	Errors affecting sound classes
Stage 4	5 yrs and older	Errors affecting late-acquired consonants, consonant clusters, and unstressed syllables in more difficult multisyllabic words

Just How Divergent Are Children?

Just how divergent are children from each other? It depends somewhat on your perspective. Where one clinician may see amazing similarities between children of the same age and level of articulation and phonological development, another clinician may see amazing differences. Many exercises in this chapter provide you the opportunity to study the speech of several children of the same age. One issue to consider as you perform these exercises is just how similar and different these children are from each other.

Stage 2

This stage occurs in typically developing toddlers from approximately 12 to 24 months of age. During this stage speech gradually comes to replace eye contact, gestures, and vocalizations as the primary means of communication as the child develops a small expressive vocabulary (typically less than 100 words by 24 months of age in typically developing toddlers) to express his or her thoughts, feelings, and needs. Articulation and phonological care of clients in this developmental stage focuses primarily on facilitating the acquisition of sounds and syllables in specific words.

Stage 3

This stage occurs in typically developing preschoolers from approximately 2 to 5 years of age. Speech is well established by the beginning of this stage, al-

though the child continues to experience difficulty in pronouncing entire sound classes. Articulation and phonological care of clients in this developmental stage focuses primarily on eliminating errors affecting sound classes.

Stage 4

This stage occurs in typically developing school-aged children approximately 5 years and older. During this stage the child's speech is similar to that of his or her community, although errors on late-acquired consonants, consonant clusters, and unstressed syllables in more difficult multisyllabic words may still occur. Articulation and phonological care of clients in this developmental stage focuses primarily on eliminating errors affecting individual consonants and consonant clusters and on producing unstressed syllables in more difficult multisyllabic words.

CHAPTER
5

Phonetic Inventories

Analysis of phonetic inventories is performed with children in Stage 2 and early Stage 3. The analysis describes a child's ability to pronounce distinctive features, sounds, syllables, and stress patterns. The analysis does not specify whether or not children speak "correctly." A phonetic inventory analysis, for example, might indicate a child's consonant inventory contains [t], [k], and [s], but would not indicate whether [t] was produced for [t] in *two* or for [z] in *zebra*.

Age norms exist for phonetic inventories of consonants. Consonant inventories based only on children's intelligible utterances are presented in Table 5–1 (Stoel-Gammon, 1985), and consonant inventories based both on intelligible and unintelligible utterances are presented in Table 5–2 (Robb & Bleile, 1994). The information in Table 5–2 is based on an experimental study (n = 7) and, consequently, should be used with some caution. The developmental level of the child's consonant inventory is that most closely approximating the number and type of the client's established consonants. For an analysis restricted only to intelligible words, a consonant is considered established when it occurs in at least two different words (the criterion used in the original studies). For an analysis of both intelligible and unintelligible words, a consonant is considered established when it occurs in at least three different words (the criterion used in the original study).

TABLE 5–1. Typical consonant inventories in children 15 through 29 months of age based on analysis of intelligible utterances.

Age	Position	Number of Consonants	Typical Consonants
15 mos*	Initial	3	b d h
	Final	none	—
18 mos*	Initial	6	b d m n h w
	Final	1	t
24 mos*	Initial	11	b d g t k m n h w f s
	Final	6	p t k n r s
29 mos**	Initial	14	b d g p t k m n h w j f s l
	Final	11	d p t k m n ŋ f s ʃ tʃ

* = Compiled from "Phonetic Inventories, 15–24 months: A Longitudinal Study," by C. Stoel-Gammon, 1985, *Journal of Speech and Hearing Research, 28*, 505–512.

** = Compiled from "Phonetic Inventories of 2- and 3-Year-old children," by A. Dyson, 1988, *Journal of Speech and Hearing Disorders, 53*, 89–93.

TABLE 5–2. Typical consonant inventories in children 12 through 24 months of age based on analysis of both intelligible and unintelligible utterances.

Age	Position	Number of Consonants	Typical Consonants
12 mos	Initial	5	b d g m h
	Final	1	m
18 mos	Initial	6	b d m n h w
	Final	2	t s
24 mos	Initial	10	b d p t k m n h s w
	Final	4	t k n s

Compiled from "Consonant Inventories of Young Children From 8 to 25 Months," by M. Robb & K. Bleile, 1994, *Journal of Clinical Linguistics and Phonetics, 8*, 295–320.

What Happened To . . . ?

It is natural to read about a young child's speech and to wonder what happened later in the child's life. Information on a child's subsequent development is included in this book whenever possible.

Exercise 5–1: Phonetic Inventories

Sometime near 1 year of age children begin using words to communicate. This exercise focuses on typical patterns and individual differences in the first words of two children, Leslie and Judy, both of whom are 11 months of age (Bleile, 1995; Ferguson, Peizer, & Weeks, 1973). For this and the other exercises in this section, consider an aspect of speech (for example, types of stress patterns) to be within a child's phonetic inventory if it occurs in two or more words, the criterion established by Stoel-Gammon for intelligible words (Stoel-Gammon, 1985). This exercise presents more diverse questions than others in the book to help you become familiar with the concepts and terminology introduced in the first section.

Judy

Judy is a happy child of 22 months with an expressive vocabulary of several hundred words. She speaks in single words and short two- to four-word sentences.

SPEECH SAMPLES

Intended Words	Leslie
1. daddy	dædæ
2. mommy	mama
3. doggie	gaga
4. patty (cake)	bæbæ

Intended Words	Judy
1. mommy	mʌm
2. daddy	da
3. yeah	ja

QUESTIONS

1. What stress patterns occur in each of the children's phonetic inventories? (**Hint:** To answer questions about phonetic inventories, cover the intended words with your hand and only look at the children's pronunciations. Also, remember to only include an aspect of speech in a child's phonetic inventory if it occurs in two or more words.) *This is an example and is answered for you.*

2. What syllable sequences occur in the words in the children's phonetic inventories? (**Hint:** This question asks you to describe words in terms of syllable boundaries and sequences of consonants and vowels. For example, the syllable sequence of the nonsense word *mumi* is CV.CV. For this and the following question, review Chapter 3, if needed.)

3. What syllable structures occur in the children's phonetic inventories? (**Hint:** This question asks you to describe two levels of syllable structure: the syllable level and the consonant and vowel level.) For example, the following is the syllable structure of the nonsense word *mumi*:

4. What consonants occur in the children's phonetic inventories? (**Hint:** Review Chapter 2, if needed.)

5. What vowels occur in the children's phonetic inventories? (**Hint:** Review Chapter 2, if needed.)

6. What distinctive features for consonants occur in the children's phonetic inventories? (**Hint:** Review Chapter 1, if needed.)

7. What distinctive features for vowels occur in the children's phonetic inventories? (**Hint:** Review Chapter 1, if needed.)

8. Summarize your answers to the above questions by describing similarities and differences in the phonetic inventories of these two 11-month-old children.

Answer Sheet for Exercise 5–1: Phonetic Inventories

1. **Stress patterns:** Leslie's words are all stressed on the first syllable and the second syllable is unstressed. Judy's words are all single syllables (and, therefore, are stressed).

2. **Leslie:** C'V . CV
   Judy: CV

3. **Leslie:** S < V C
   Judy: S < V C

4. **Leslie:** no consonants
   Judy: no consonants   ✓

5. **Leslie:** ~~a~~ a → æ
   Judy: a

6. **Leslie:** all consonants are voiced, bilabial → oral stops
   Judy: all consonants are voiced

7. **Leslie:** vowels are front, [a] is open, [æ] is between mid & open
   Judy: vowel is front

8. **Similarities:** CV syllable structures, the vowel [a] & voicing for consonants

9. **Differences:** stress patterns, [æ] only in Leslie

Exercise 5–2: Phonetic Inventories

This and the following exercise provide opportunities to see how phonetic inventories develop between approximately 15 to 24 months of age, the age range during which that type of analysis is chiefly used. For the present exercise, describe the phonetic inventories of Davie and a child (no name is given in the article in which the child's speech is described) who are 15 and 16 months of age, respectively (Bleile, 1995; Branigan, 1976). The questions focus on the phonetic inventories of syllables and consonants, both of which are critical to understanding typical development and also play crucial roles in the evaluation and treatment of clients with articulation and phonological disorders.

Davie

Davie is a kindly child of 26 months with an expressive vocabulary of many hundreds of words. He speaks in short sentences.

SPEECH SAMPLES

Intended Words	Davie
1. book	bʊ
2. binky	bi
3. up	ʌp
4. juice	dʒu
5. that	ʃat
6. momma	mɑmʌ́
7. daddy	dadá~
	dádá
8. down	daʊn
9. balloon	jun
10. pop	ɑp
11. ball	bɔ
12. hot	hat
13. shoe	ʃu
14. cookies	koʊkoʊ́
15. baby	beɪbí
16. mine	maɪn
17. apple	apʊ́~
	ápʊ
18. key	ki

Intended Words	Child
1. eye	eɪ
2. goose	gu
3. hi	ha
4. bye	ba

(continued)

Intended Words	Child
(continued)	
5. kitty	ki
6. button	bʌ
7. mouth	maʊ
8. clock	ta
9. dog	wuwu
10. daddy	dada
11. no-no	nunu
12. popcorn	pap pap

QUESTIONS

1. What consonants occur in each child's word final phonetic inventories? (**Hint:** As with Exercise 5–1, do not be concerned whether or not a syllable or consonant is produced correctly and only place a consonant or syllable in a child's phonetic inventory if it occurs in two or more words.) *This is an example and is answered for you.*

2. Which syllable sequences occur in each child's phonetic inventory?

3. Complete the table on the answer sheet to show which possible noncluster syllable structures occur in the phonetic inventory of each child. *The first part of this question is an example and is answered for you.*

4. According to the developmental age norms in Table 5–1, which and how many word initial consonants typically occur in the speech of children 15 months of age? Which and how many word initial consonants occur in the speech of each child?

5. Complete the table on the answer sheet showing which manners of production typically occur in the speech of children near 15 months of age (Table 5–1) and which occur in word initial position in the speech of each child. *The first part of this question is an example and is answered for you.*

6. As with the fifth question, complete the table on the answer sheet showing which places of production typically occur in the speech of children near 15 months of age (Table 5–1) and which occur in word initial position in the speech of each child.

7. Answer the following questions about common characteristics in development based on your answers to the previous questions.

    A. Which syllable structure or syllable structures occur in the speech of both children?
    B. Which word initial consonant or consonants occur in the speech of both children?
    C. Which manner or manners of production occur in word initial position in the speech of both children?
    D. Which place or places of production occur in word initial position in the speech of both children?

8. Answer the following questions about individual differences in consonant development based on your answers to the previous questions.

    A. Which consonants typically occur in the word initial consonant inventories of children near 15 months of age according to developmental age norms? Which consonants occur in the speech of each of the two children? *This is an example and is answered for you.*
    B. How many consonants typically occur in the word initial consonant inventories of children near 15 months of age according to developmental age norms? How many occur in the speech of each of the two children?
    C. Which manners of production typically occur in the word initial consonant inventories of children near 15 months of age according to developmental age norms? Which occur in the speech of each of the two children?
    D. Which places of production typically occur in the word initial consonant inventories of children near 15 months of age according to developmental age norms? Which occur in the speech of each of the two children?

Answer Sheet for Exercise 5–2: Phonetic Inventories

1. **Davie:** n t p
   Child: none

2. **Davie:**
   Child:

3.

Children	V	CV	CVC	VC
Davie:		✓		
Child:				

4. **Table 5–1:**
   Davie:
   Child:

5.

Children	Stops	Nasals	Fricatives	Affricates	Glides	Liquids
Table 5–1:	✓					
Davie:						
Child:						

6.

Children	Bi.	LabD.	InterD.	Al.	PostA.	Pal.	Vel.	Glot.
Table 5–1:								
Davie:								
Child:								

7. A. **Syllable structure:**
   B. **Consonant:**
   C. **Manner of production:**
   D. **Place of production:**

8. A. **Types of consonants:** Norms = b d h
   Davie = b d k m ʃ
   Child = b

B. **Number of consonants:** Norms =

Davie =

Child =

C. **Manners of production:** Norms =

Davie =

Child =

D. **Places of production:**   Norms =

Davie =

Child =

Exercise 5–3: Phonetic Inventories

The analysis of phonetic inventories, so useful with children in Stage 2, becomes increasingly less valuable as children's expressive vocabularies expand to include an increasingly wide range of stress patterns, sequences of syllables, types of syllables, consonants, vowels, and distinctive features. For this exercise, describe the word initial consonant inventories of four children, each of whom are 2 years of age. Each child is in early Stage 3, which is near the maximum point at which analysis of phonetic inventories is used.

Hildegard

My information about Hildegard is second hand and several years old. I was told at that time that Hildegard, the little girl who had said *pillow* as [bi] and *spoon* as [bu], was now a proud grandmother.

Amahl

Amahl has come full circle. The subject of a famous linguistic study is now a linguist.

SPEECH SAMPLE

See Appendix B–1 through B–4.

QUESTIONS

1. What consonants occur in Hildegard's word initial phonetic inventory? (**Hint:** Remember that for this analysis you are interested in the child's capacity to produce consonants, not whether the consonants are produced correctly. Also, for this exercise do not count consonants in consonant clusters and, as previously, only place a consonant in a child's phonetic inventory if it occurs in two or more words.) *This is an example and is answered for you.*

2. According to the developmental age norms in Table 5–1, which consonants typically occur in word initial position in children near 24 months of age? Which word initial consonants occur in the phonetic invento-

ries of Hildegard, Kylie, Amahl, and Jake? (*Hint:* For the purpose of this exercise, do not count glottal stops in the phonetic inventories.)

3. According to the developmental age norms in Table 5–1, how many consonants typically occur in word initial position in children near 24 months of age? How many word initial consonants occur in the speech of each of the four children?

4. According to the developmental age norms in Table 5–1, which manners of production typically occur in the word initial consonants in children near 24 months of age? Perform the same analysis for each of the 4 children. *The first part of this question is an example and is answered for you.*

5. According to the developmental age norms in Table 5–1, which places of production typically occur in the word initial consonants in children near 24 months of age? Perform the same analysis for each of these four children.

6. Summarize your answers to the above questions to better see the typical patterns and individual differences in the word initial consonant inventories of children near 24 months of age.

    A. Which word initial consonants typically occur in the speech of children near 24 months of age? Which of the 4 children have this typical consonant inventory?

    B. What is the average number of word initial consonants in the speech of children near 24 months of age? What range occurs in the speech of the four children?

    C. What manners of production typically occur in word initial position in the speech of children near 24 months of age? What range of manners of production occur in the speech of the four children? *This is an example and is answered for you.*

    D. What places of production typically occur in word initial position in the speech of children near 24 months of age? What range of places of production occur in the speech of the 4 children?

7. *For discussion:* Why do you suppose analyses of sounds pronounced correctly is seldom undertaken with children in Stage 2?

Answer Sheet for Exercise 5–3: Phonetic Inventories

1. **Hildegard:** p t b d g m n h j w

2. **Table 5–1:** b d g t k m n h w f s
   Hildegard: p t b d g m n f ʃ h w
   Kylie: p t b d m n
   Amahl: p b d m n
   Jake: p t b d g m n f ð dʒ

3. **Table 5–1:** 11
   Hildegard: 10
   Kylie: 12
   Amahl: 8
   Jake: 15

4.

Children	Stops	Nasals	Fricatives	Affricates	Glides	Liquids
Table 5–1:	✓					
Hildegard:						
Kylie:						
Amahl:						
Jake:						

5.

Children	Bi.	LabD.	InterD.	Al.	PostA.	Pal.	Vel.	Glot.
Table 5–1:								
Hildegard:								
Kylie:								
Amahl:								
Jake:								

6. A. **Typical consonant inventory:** t k b d g m n f s h w

    Child with typical inventory: none

  B. **Average:** 11

    Range: 9 to 15

  C. **Typical:** stops, nasals, fricatives, and glides

    Range: Hildegard has the fewest number of different manners of production in her consonant inventory (stops, nasals, glides). Jake has the greatest number of different manners of production in his consonant inventory (stops, nasals, fricatives, an affricate, and glides.)

  D. **Typical:** bilabial, labiodental, alveolar, velar t glottal

    Range: Amahl has smallest # places of production. Jake has greatest #

7. *For discussion:*

Children in this stage produce most sounds incorrectly

Exercise 5–4: Phonetic Inventories

This exercise provides a means to summarize what you've learned about typical patterns and individual differences in word initial consonant inventories between 15 and 24 months, the period during which phonetic inventory analysis is of the greatest benefit. Base the summary on your answers to Exercises 5–2 and 5–3.

QUESTIONS

1. Which word initial consonants typically occur in the speech of children at 15 and at 24 months of age according to developmental age norms? Which word initial consonants occur in the speech of one or both

of the children at 15 months of age and which occur in the speech of two or more of the children at 24 months of age?

2. How many word initial consonants typically occur in the speech of children at 15 and at 24 months of age according to developmental age norms? What is the range of number of word initial consonants for the children at each of those ages?

3. Which manners of production occur in word initial position at 15 and at 24 months of age according to developmental age norms? Which manners of production occur in the speech of one or both the children 15 months of age, and which manners of production occur in the speech of two or more of the children at 24 months of age?

4. Which places of production occur in word initial position at 15 and at 24 months of age according to developmental age norms? Which places of production occur in the speech of one or both the children 15 months of age, and which places of production occur in the speech of two or more of the children at 24 months of age?

Answer Sheet for Exercise 5–4

1.

Consonants	15 Months	24 Months
Norms:	b d n	
Children:	b d k m j	

2.

Number of Consonants	15 Months	24 Months
Norms:	3	11
Children:	1 to 5	a to 15

3.

Manners	15 Months	24 Months
Norms:	stops & glides	stops, glides nasals fric.
Children:	stops, nasals fricatives	11 11

4.

Places	15 Months	24 Months
Norms:	bilabial, alveolar	
Children:	bilabial alveolar velar	

CHAPTER
6

Error Patterns

An error pattern analysis is performed with children in Stages 2 and 3. The analysis describes errors affecting two or more sounds. Error patterns encompass both what are traditionally called phonological processes as well as certain types of articulation errors. The term error pattern is used in this book to avoid biasing the discussion toward either an articulation or phonological perspective. The appendix of this chapter contains definitions of 23 common and uncommon error patterns.

Exercise 6–1: Error Patterns

The exercises in this section consider error patterns in the speech of children without articulation and phonological disorders. Similar error patterns are found in the speech of clients with articulation and phonological disorders. The exercises are arranged in roughly chronological order. The first exercise considers an error pattern that affects stress in multisyllabic words in the speech of Davie, the child 15 months of age whose phonetic inventory was analyzed in the previous chapter.

SPEECH SAMPLE

Intended Words	Davie
1. book	bʊ
2. binky	bi
3. up	ʌp
4. juice	dʒu

(continued)

SPEECH SAMPLE *(continued)*

Intended Words	Davie
5. that	ʃat
6. mamma	mɑmʌ́
7. daddy	dadá– dádá
8. down	daʊn
9. balloon	jun
10. pop	ɑp
11. ball	bɔ
12. hot	hat
13. shoe	ʃu
14. cookies	koʊkoʊ́
15. baby	beɪbí
16. mine	maɪn
17. apple	apú́– ápʊ
18. key	ki

QUESTIONS

1. What does the slash above a vowel indicate? (**Hint:** If needed, see the appendix of Chapter 4.)

2. Identify which of Davie's words are multisyllabic.

3. On which syllable does primary stress fall in these words? If there are exceptions to this pattern, be sure to note them.

4. Compare the syllable on which primary stress falls in Davie's speech to where it falls in the words on the left. Based on this comparison, describe Davie's error pattern.

5. Think of your answer to question 3 as an initial hypothesis. To test your hypothesis, describe a method to teach Davie to say *happy* and *bubble*. If your hypothesis is correct, how will Davie pronounce stress in these words?

6. *For discussion:* It seems fairly certain that people with whom Davie was in contact did not pronounce words such as *mamma, daddy, cookies,* and *baby* with primary stress on the second syllable. Nor do words with primary stress on the second syllable occur earlier in development than words with primary stress on the first syllable, so Davie's error pattern is not equivalent to substituting an earlier acquired stress pattern for a later one. Think a while about the problem posed by Davie's unusual error pattern and try to develop some hypotheses about how such an error pattern might have come about.

Answer Sheet for Exercise 6–1: Error Patterns

1. **Slash:**

2. **Multisyllabic:**

3. **Primary stress:**

4. **Error pattern:**

5. *Happy* **and** *bubble:*

6. *For discussion:*

Exercise 6–2: Error Patterns

This exercise considers two error patterns, one affecting consonants and the other vowels. The exercise is based on the speech of a child named Jacob from between 1 year, 6 months to 1 year, 9 months of age (Menn, 1976).

Jacob*

Jacob is a talented young man with interests in sculpture and child care.

SPEECH SAMPLE

Intended Words	Jacob*
1. tape	ti
2. duck	dʌ
3. close	doʊ
4. okay	ki
5. gate	gi
6. whee	i
7. cow	kaʊ
8. "A"	i
9. cake	gik˜
	keɪk

*The following words are exceptions to the error pattern: *away, lady, Jacob, rain.*

QUESTION

1. What is the name of the error pattern that affects Jacob's pronunciation of words ending in consonants?

2. Which of the 10 words is an exception to the above error pattern?

3. List two words that you could teach Jacob to test if your hypothesis about this error pattern is correct.

4. Now consider Jacob's other error pattern. To begin, use the x – y notation (see Chapter 4) to list Jacob's vowel errors. *The first part of this question is an example and is answered for you.*

5. Based on your answer to the fourth question, which vowel is pronounced as [i]?

6. Describe Jacob's vowel error pattern using distinctive features.

7. If your hypothesis is correct, how would Jacob pronounce the vowels in *hay* and *duke*?

Answer Sheet for Exercise 6–2: Error Patterns

1. **Error pattern:**

2. **Exception:**

3. **Possible words:**

4. **Words:**
   1. tape [eɪ] – [i]

5. **Affected vowel:**

6. **Distinctive features:**

7. *hay* **and** *duke*:

Exercise 6–3: Error Patterns

Error patterns resulting from assimilations are common in the speech of many younger children. The speech of the following child contains two common assimilation patterns that interact with each other in interesting ways. The assimilation patterns occur in the child's speech from between 1 year, 6 months to 1 year, 10 months of age (Cruttenden, 1978).

SPEECH SAMPLE

Intended Words	Child
1. doggie	gʊgi
2. cuddle	kʊku
3. rabbit	babi
4. man	mam
5. crispies	pipi
6. piggy	pɪpi
7. apple	papa
8. about*	bəbaʊ
9. all gone	gʊgʊn
10. acorn*	kɛkʊn

*These words were not spoken by the child, but follow his pattern. I added the words to provide additional examples for the exercise.

QUESTIONS

1. Words 1 and 2 are examples of a common assimilation pattern. What is the name of the pattern?

2. Words 3 and 4 are examples of another common assimilation pattern. What is the name of the pattern?

3. What is the place of production of the consonants that assimilated in words 1 through 4?

4. Words such as 5 and 6 contain both labial and velar consonants. Did Velar Assimilation or Labial Assimilation occur?

5. Develop a hypothesis that describes the error patterns and interactions between error patterns in words 1 through 6.

6. How does your hypothesis predict that the child will pronounce the consonants in the following words? *The first part of this question is an example and is answered for you.*

   A. dig
   B. bug
   C. pit
   D. tub

7. The words (a phrase in one instance) 7 through 10 begin with vowels in the adult language, but are produced with initial consonants by the child. Notice each word begins with a different consonant. What determines which consonant begins words 7 through 10? (**Hint:** Ignore the [l] in *all gone*, which the child may not have heard because it is not pronounced by many speakers.)

8. List two words that you might teach the child to determine if your hypothesis is correct. Indicate which sound you think the child will pronounce at the beginning of each word.

Answer Sheet for Exercise 6–3: Error Patterns

1. **Error pattern:**

2. **Error pattern:**

3. **Place of production:**

4. **Assimilation:**

5. **Hypothesis:**

6. A. g g
   B.
   C.
   D.

7. **Hypothesis:**

8. **Possible words:**

Exercise 6–4: Error Patterns

In most cases, consonants assimilate to other consonants, as with Labial Assimilation and Velar Assimilation. However, consonants can also assimilate to vowels, especially among children in earlier stages of articulation and phonological development. The speech of the child that is the focus of this exercise contains such an error pattern (Braine, 1974; Stoel-Gammon, 1983). The exercise focuses on an assimilation pattern in the child's speech from between 20 to 23 months of age.

Assimilation

A primary reason to transcribe the entire word of younger children is that the occurrence of a sound in one part of a word may influence that in another part of a word. To illustrate, a child may regularly pronounce [k] as [t] through Fronting (for example, the child may pronounce *key* as [ti]), but may say [k] as [p] in words such as *keep* through Labial Assimilation. If the whole word is not transcribed, the clinician is not able to explain why sometimes [k] is pronounced as [t] and other times as [p].

The most common types of assimilations are relatively few in number; although, of course, less frequent types of assimilations may also occur. Consonants that cause consonants to assimilate are described elsewhere in this book (see Labial Assimilation and Velar Assimilation). The following are the "best bets" when it is suspected that a vowel is causing a consonant to assimilate:

- Front vowels (especially [i]) may cause a nearby consonant to assimilate to the alveolar place of production (example: *key* as [ti]). This is because front vowels are produced only slightly back in the mouth from where alveolar consonants are produced.
- Back vowels (especially [u]) may cause a nearby consonant to assimilate to the velar place of production (example: *two* as [ku]. This is because back vowels and velar consonants are produced near the same place in the back of the mouth.
- A vowel may cause a preceding consonant to be voiced (example: *pea* as [bi]). This is because the vowel is voiced. Rather than producing the consonant without voicing and then turning on the voicing, the consonant and vowel are both produced with voicing.
- Vowels preceding and following a voiceless consonant (called an **intervocalic consonant**) may cause the consonant to be voiced (example: the nonsense word [isi] being pronounced [izi]). As above, this is because the vowels are voiced, and the change makes it possible to "turn on" voicing for all three sounds, rather than turning on voicing for the first vowel, turning it off for the consonant, and then turning it on again for the vowel.

SPEECH SAMPLE

Intended Words	Child
1. ball	bɔ.ʊ
2. mama	mama
3. pad*	pæ
4. big	dɪʔ
5. boo*	bu
6. milk	nɪʔ
7. bʌbʌbʌbi**	babadi
8. me*	ni
9. pa*	pa
10. "B"	dɪʔ

*= Words followed by * are added to better illustrate the child's error pattern.

**= a nonsense word that the child imitates

QUESTIONS

1. How many syllable initial consonant errors occur in these 10 words? (*Hint:* Remember that each consonant in word 7 is in syllable initial position.) *This is an example and is answered for you.*

2. Describe the place of production changes in syllable initial consonants.

3. Consider the consonants produced in error. Which vowels follow these consonants?

4. Develop a hypothesis that describes this child's error pattern.

5. How does your hypothesis suggest the child will pronounce the first consonants in *meet, bit,* and *bat*?

6. Suppose a colleague believes that your hypothesis is incorrect and hypothesizes instead that the error pattern is caused by all close vowels. Which of the 10 words could be used to argue against this alternative hypothesis? Why?

Answer Sheet for Exercise 6–4: Error Patterns

1. **Syllable initial consonants:** 5

2. **Place of production change:**

3. **Vowels:**

4. **Hypothesis:**

5. *Meet, bit,* **and** *bat:*

6. **Alternative hypothesis:**

Exercise 6–5: Error Patterns

This exercise focuses on a somewhat unusual error pattern in the speech of a child aged from between approximately 1 year, 9 months to 2 years, 2 months of age (Fey & Gandour, 1982). The error pattern influences consonants in the ends of words.

SPEECH SAMPLE

Intended Words	Child
1. big	bigŋ̩
2. egg	ɛgŋ̩
3. read	widn̩
4. drop	dap
5. stub	dabm̩
6. eat	it
7. word	wʊdn̩
8. talk	dɔk
9. lightbulb	jaɪtbabm̩
10. fit	vɪt

QUESTIONS

1. What is the meaning of the line under the nasal consonant in the first word? (*Hint:* If needed, see the appendix of Chapter 4.)

2. Which class of sounds is added to the end of certain words?

3. Sometimes [m] is added to a word and other times [n] or the velar nasal is added. Develop a hypothesis that describes which consonant is added.

4. Suppose you decide to teach the child some new words. According to your hypothesis, which consonant will be added to *mud* and *bib*?

5. Notice that an additional consonant is not added to certain words. Develop a hypothesis that explains why. (*Hint:* The words are not exceptions.)

6. According to your hypothesis, will a consonant be added to words ending in [k]? If your answer is yes, indicate which consonant will be added.

Answer Sheet for Exercise 6–5: Error Patterns

1. **Diacritic:**

2. **Sound class:**

3. **Hypothesis:**

4. *Mud* **and** *bib*:

5. **Hypothesis:**

6. **Words ending in [k]:**

Exercise 6–6: Error Patterns

This exercise focuses on an error pattern in the speech of Kylie, a child 2 years of age (Bleile, 1987).

SPEECH SAMPLE

Intended Words	Kylie
171. lion	jaɪ.ɪn
172. lamby	læmi
173. leg	jɛg
174. lawnmower	jæmaʊ
175. robin	wɑbɪn
176. read	wi
177. rabbit	wæbɪt
178. rabbits	wæbɪs
179. raccoon	wækun
180. ring	wiŋ
181. rock (n)	wɑk

QUESTIONS

1. Which manner of production includes [l r], but not [w j]?

2. What is the name of the error pattern that affects Kylie's pronunciation of word initial [l r]?

3. One word is an exception to the error pattern affecting [l]. What is the word?

4. Suppose Kylie had pronounced [l] and [r] as [w]. What would the error pattern be called?

5. Suppose Kylie had pronounced [l] and [r] as [d]. (It's not a common error pattern, but it occurs.) What would the error pattern be called?

6. Sometimes a special notation provides a convenient means to describe error patterns. Use the notation x – y/z (see Chapter 4) to state that liquids are pronounced as glides in word initial position.

Answer Sheet for Error 6–6: Error Patterns

1. **Manner of production:**

2. **Error pattern:**

3. **Exception:**

4. **Error pattern:**

5. **Error pattern:**

6. **Notation:**

Exercise 6–7: Error Patterns

More than one error pattern may affect the same word. Similarly, multiple error patterns may affect consonants belonging to the same sound class. This exercise focuses on two error patterns that occur in the speech of a child named Hildegard at 2 years of age (Leopold, 1947).

SPEECH SAMPLE

Intended Words	Hildegard
1. pillow	bi
2. piece	bis
3. peas	bi
4. piano	ba
5. papa	baba
6. pail	be.a
7. pick	bɪt
8. put	bʊ
9. paper	bubu
10. pudding	bʊ.ɪ
11. push	bʊʃ
12. poor	pu
13. pretty	pɪti
14. please	bis
15. towel	daʊ
16. toast	dok
17. too	du

(continued)

SPEECH SAMPLE *(continued)*

Intended Words	Hildegard
18. toothbrush	tuʃbaʃ
19. two	tu
20. train	te
21. cover	da
22. candy	da.i
23. kiss	dɪʃ
24. cold	do
25. comb	do
26. coat	dot~ nʊk
27. cake	gek
28. cookies	tutiʃ
29. cry	daɪ
30. crash	daʃ
31. cracker	gaga

QUESTIONS

1. What error pattern affects most of Hildegard's words that begin with [p] and [t]?

2. Which words beginning with [p] and [t] are exceptions to this error pattern?

3. More than one error pattern can affect the same word. Many words beginning with initial [k] are affected by both Prevocalic Voicing and Fronting. What are those words? (**Hint:** Because a number of words are affected, it is easier to list the word numbers rather than writing each word.)

4. Which words beginning with [k] are pronounced with Prevocalic Voicing, but not Fronting?

5. Which word beginning with [k] is pronounced with Fronting, but not Prevocalic Voicing?

6. Hildegard's pronunciation of *coat* with a word initial [n] could have resulted from a relatively uncommon error pattern. What is the name of that pattern?

7. Use the notation x → y/z (see Chapter 4) to state that voiceless oral stops are voiced in the beginning of words.

Answer Sheet for Exercise 6–7: Error Patterns

1. **Error pattern:**

2. **Exceptions:**

3. **Word numbers:**

4. **Words:**

5. **Word:**

6. **Error pattern:**

7. **Notation:**

Exercise 6–8: Error Patterns

Although a child's pronunciation of a word occasionally contains error patterns one day and no error patterns the next, most often improvement occurs over months and, in some cases, years, especially among clients with articulation and phonological disorders. This exercise shows how a child named Amahl learns to pronounce 2 words from between 2 years, 3 months to 3 years, 0 months of age (Smith, 1973).

SPEECH SAMPLE

Intended Words	Amahl	Approx. Age
driving	1. waɪbɪn	2;3
	2. daɪvɪn	2;5
	3. draɪvɪn	2;7
sauce	1. dɔd	2;4
	2. dɔt	2;5
	3. tʰɔt	2;8
	4. tɔt~	2;11
	tsɔts~	
	sɔts	
	5. sɔs	3;0

QUESTIONS

1. Which two common error patterns affect Amahl's pronunciation of word initial [dr] in *driving* at 2 years, 3 months of age?

2. Complete the table showing how Amahl gradually overcame error patterns affecting his pronunciation of *driving*. (**Hint:** All the error patterns are common and are listed in the appendix to this chapter).

3. Which two common error patterns affect Amahl's pronunciation of word initial [s] in sauce at 2 years, 4 months of age?

4. Two error patterns affect Amahl's pronunciation of [s] in word final position at 2 years, 4 months of age. One is common and the other somewhat unusual. Identify the common error pattern and describe the unusual one (it hasn't a name).

5. Complete the table to show how Amahl gradually learns to pronounce *sauce*. (**Hint:** All the error patterns are listed in the appendix of this chapter, although not all are common.)

Answer Sheet for Exercise 6–8: Error Patterns

1. **Error patterns:**
2.

driving

Ages	Word Initial Position	Intervocalic Position
1. 2;3		
2. 2;5		
3. 2;7		

3. **Word initial error patterns:**
4. **Word final error patterns:**
5.

sauce

Ages	Word Initial Position	Word Final Position
1. 2;4		
2. 2;5		
3. 2;8		
3. 2;11	(1)	
	(2)	
	(3)	
5. 3;0		

Exercise 6–9: Error Patterns

By their third year of life, many children pronounce stops, nasals, and glides correctly in isolated words, although errors may still occur occasionally in consonant clusters, longer words, and sentences. Children in their third year of life may continue to have difficulties pronouncing certain fricatives and liquids in all contexts. This exercise shows an error pattern of a 3 year, 6 month old child named Rikki (see Appendix B-6 for the complete speech sample).

SPEECH SAMPLE

Intended Words	Rikki
26. crab	kwæb
27. crayon	kwæn
28. clown	kwaʊn
29. clock	kəlɑk
42. bridge	bwɪdʒ
43. broom	bwum

(continued)

SPEECH SAMPLE *(continued)*

Intended Words	Rikki
47. drum	dʒwʌm
51. grass	græs
52. glass	glæs~
	gəlæs
64. french fries	fwɛntʃ fwaɪz
65. frog	fwɑg
66. flag	fwæg
78. strawberry	ʃtrɔbɛwi
79. string	ʃtrɪŋ
82. sled	slɛd
90. choo choo	tʃutʃu
train	tʃweɪn
107. radio	weɪdi.oʊ
108. rose	woʊs
109. rain	weɪn
110. rocket ship	wɑkɪn ʃɪp
111. rope	woʊp
112. lamp	læmp
113. lemon	lɛmɪn
114. letter	lɛɾi
115. lion	laɪn
116. lettuce	lɛɾɪs
117. leaf	lif
118. lunch	lʌntʃ

QUESTIONS

1. What error pattern affects the greatest number of words beginning with [l] and [r]?

2. Another error pattern affects Rikki's pronunciation of consonant clusters in words 29 and 52. What is the name of that error pattern?

3. The error patterns affecting [r] has exceptions. In which phonetic environment (next to a vowel or in consonant clusters) is [r] more likely to be produced correctly?

4. List the words in which [r] is produced correctly.

5. It seems somewhat surprising that [r] is produced correctly in consonant clusters with [g] and [st], but not in other consonant clusters. Although it may be that [g] and [st] are key environments for Rikki, another possibility is that more complete sampling would reveal other consonant clusters in which Rikki could produce [r]. To test these hypotheses, list 3 words you could use to determine if Rikki can pronounce [r] in [kr] consonant clusters.

6. The error patterns affecting [l] also has exceptions. In which phonetic environment (next to a vowel or in consonant clusters) is [l] more likely to be produced correctly?

7. In which consonant clusters is [l] pronounced correctly?

8. As with [r], although it may be that [gl] and [sl] are facilitating contexts for Rikki, another possibility is that more complete sampling would reveal other consonant clusters in which Rikki could produce [l]. Illustrate the latter hypothesis by listing three words you could use to determine if Rikki can pronounce [l] in [fl] consonant clusters.

Answer Sheet for Exercise 6–9: Error Patterns

1. **Error pattern:**

2. **Error pattern:**

3. **Phonetic environment:**

4. **Words:**

5. **[kr] consonant clusters:**

6. **Phonetic environment:**

7. **Consonant clusters:**

8. **[fl] consonant cluster:**

Exercise 6–10: Error Patterns

By 5 years of age children's speech errors most often affect individual sounds rather than sound classes. A child whose speech contained Gliding when he or she was 3 years of age, for example, may show [w] coloring of [r] when 5 years of age. Similarly, a child whose speech contained Lisping error patterns when he or she was 4 years of age, may still lisp [s] at 5 years of age when tired or excited. An exception to the general rule that speech errors only affect individual sounds at this stage occurs in longer words with relatively unfamiliar stress patterns. The speech of the child who is the focus of this exercise contains such an error pattern (Izuka, 1995).

SPEECH SAMPLE

Intended Words	Ryan
1. telescope	tɛləskoʊp
2. refrigerator	frɪdʒɚ.eɪɾɚ
3. alphabet	aʊlfəbɛt
4. astronomy	ʃranɑmi
5. ice skate	aɪs skeɪt
6. iambic	jɑmbɪk
7. barbarian	bɑbeɪri.ɛn
8. hop scotch	hɑp skɑtʃ
9. revolutionize	rɛvoʊluʃənaɪz
10. see saw	sisɔ
11. astrological	æʃtroʊlɑdʒɪkl̩
12. concomitant	kəkɑmɪntɪnt
13. teeter totter	tiɾɚ tɑɾɚ
14. memory	mɛmɔri
15. vaccination	væksɪneɪʃn̩

QUESTIONS

1. List the numbers of the words that contain errors in their initial syllable. (**Hint**: Ignore apparent errors elsewhere in the words. The postalveolar fricative in *astronomy* and *astrological* was a dialect pattern rather than a speech error, and syllabic [l] and [n] in *astrological* and *vaccination*, respectively, occur normally in conversational speech.)

2. List the numbers of the intended words that typically receive primary stress on the second syllable. (**Hint:** Remember, for this question focus on the intended words rather than Ryan's pronunciations.)

3. Describe Ryan's error pattern based on your answers to the first two questions.

4. Ryan's error pattern appears to reflect an English bias for a certain type of stress pattern. What is the name of that stress pattern? (**Hint:** If necessary, review the exercises on stress in Chapter 3.)

5. Of the four speech errors, three involve deletion of syllables. This seems to be an advanced form of an error pattern that affects the speech of much younger children. What is the name of that error pattern?

Answer Sheet for Exercise 6–10: Error Patterns

1. **Words:**

2. **Intended words:**

3. **Error pattern:**

4. **Stress pattern:**

5. **Error pattern:**

APPENDIX

Error Patterns

Common error patterns are listed on the following page. Next, definitions of both common and uncommon error patterns are provided. The stars (***) next to a definition indicate that the error pattern occurs commonly.

List of Commonly Occurring Error Patterns

Changes in Place of Production

>   Fronting
>   Lisping
>   Labial assimilation
>   Velar assimilation

Changes in Manner of Production

>   Stopping
>   Gliding
>   Lateralization

Changes in the Beginning of Syllables or Words

>   Prevocalic voicing

Changes at the End of Syllables or Words

>   Final consonant devoicing
>   Final consonant deletion

Changes in Syllables

>   Reduplication
>   Syllable deletion

Changes in Consonant Clusters

>   Cluster reduction
>   Epenthesis (ePENthesis)

Changes in Vowels and Syllabic Consonants

Vowel neutralization
Vocalization

Definitions of Error Patterns

A. Changes in Place of Production

Fronting***: Velar consonants (and sometimes postalveolar affricates) are pronounced as alveolar consonants; for example, *key* is pronounced [ti].

Lisping***: Alveolar consonants (typically fricatives) are pronounced with the tongue either on or between the front teeth; for example, *see* is pronounced [si]. Also called a frontal lisp. Lateral lisps are the same as lisping, except the airflow comes over the sides of the tongue.

Labial assimilation***: Consonants assimilate to the place of production of a labial consonant; for example, *bead* is pronounced [bib].

Velar assimilation***: Consonants assimilate to the place of production of a velar consonant; for example, *teak* is pronounced [kik].

Backing: Alveolar consonants are replaced by velar consonants; for example, *tee* is pronounced as [ki].

Glottal replacement: A consonant is pronounced as a glottal stop; for example, *boot* is pronounced [buʔ].

B. Changes in Manner of Production

Stopping***: A sound (typically a fricative or affricate) is pronounced as an oral stop; for example, the pronunciation of *see* as [ti].

Gliding***: A liquid consonant is pronounced as a glide; for example, *Lee* is pronounced [wi] or (less typically) [ji].

Lateralization***: Sounds typically produced with central air emission (most commonly [s] and [z]) are pronounced with lateral air emission; for example, *see* is pronounce [ˌsi].

Affrication: Stops or fricatives are pronounced as affricates; for example, *see* is pronounced as [tsi].

Nasalization: Non-nasal consonants (usually oral stops) are pronounced as nasal stops; for example, *bee* is pronounced [mi].

Denasalization: Nasal consonants are pronounced as oral consonants (typically oral stops); for example, *me* is pronounced [bi].

C. Changes in the Beginning of Syllables or Words

Prevocalic voicing***: Consonants are voiced when they occur before a vowel; for example, *pea* pronounced as [bi].

Initial consonant deletion: An error pattern in which the consonant beginning a word is deleted; for example, *bee* is pronounced [i].

D. Changes at the End of Syllables or Words

Final consonant devoicing***: Voiced obstruents are devoiced at the end of a syllable or word; for example, *mead* is pronounced as [mit].

Final consonant deletion***: A consonant occurring at the end of a syllable or word is deleted; for example, *beet* is pronounced [bi].

E. Changes in Syllables

Reduplication***: A syllable is repeated; for example, the pronunciation of *water* as [wɑwɑ].
Syllable deletion***: Unstressed syllable is deleted; for example, *banana* is pronounced as [nænə].

F. Changes in Consonant Clusters

Cluster reduction***: A consonant or consonants in a consonant cluster are deleted; for example, *speed* is pronounced as [pid] or [sid].
Epenthesis (ePENthesis)***: A vowel is inserted between consonants in a consonant cluster; for example, *treat* is pronounced [tərit].

G. Sound Reversals

Metathesis (MeTAthesis): The order of sounds in a word is reversed; for example, *peek* is pronounced [kip].

H. Changes in Vowels and Syllabic Consonants

Vowel neutralization***: A vowel is replaced with a neutral vowel; for example, *bat* is pronounced [bʌt].
Vocalization***. A syllabic consonant is replaced by a neutral vowel; for example, *beetle* is pronounced [birə].

Consonants and Consonant Clusters

Analysis of consonants and consonant clusters is undertaken with children in Stages 2 through 4. This analysis describes a child's ability to produce individual consonants and consonant clusters. The ages at which consonants and consonant clusters are typically acquired are listed in Tables 7–1 and 7–2 (Smit, Hand, Frelinger, Bernthal, & Byrd, 1990). To be included in the tables, a sound needed to meet two criteria: (1) at least 50% of both males and females correctly produced the sound in word initial and word final positions (consonants) or word initial position (consonant clusters), and (2) the percentage of subjects correctly producing the sound at subsequent age levels never dropped below 50%.

Exercise 7–1: Consonants and Consonant Clusters

The consonants and consonant clusters of American English are largely acquired between a child's first and fifth birthday, even though the speech of a child over 5 years of age may continue to exhibit random speech errors and may display error patterns and errors on sounds in longer words with unfamiliar stress patterns. This exercise offers an opportunity to consider typical patterns in consonant and consonant cluster development.

TABLE 7–1. Age of acquisition (50% to 75% correct) of American English consonants averaged across both word initial and word final positions.

Consonant	50%	75%	Consonant	50%	75%
m	<3;0	<3;0	f	<3;0	3;6
n	<3;0	<3;0	v	3;6	4;6
ŋ	<3;0	7;6*	θ	4;6	6;0
h	<3;0	<3;0	ɚ	4;6	5;6
w	<3;0	<3;0	s	3;6	5;0
j	<3;0	3;6	z	4;0	6;0
p	<3;0	<3;0	ʃ	3;6	5;0
t	<3;0	<3;0	tʃ	3;6	6;0
k	<3;0	<3;0	dʒ	3;6	4;6
b	<3;0	<3;0	r	3;6	6;0
d	<3;0	<3;0	l	3;6	6;0
g	<3;0	<3;0	ð	4;6	5;6

* = Transcriber difficulties may have resulted in this sound being acquired at 7;6.

Compiled from "The Iowa Articulation Norms Project and Its Nebraska Replication," by A. Smit, L. Hand, J. Frelinger, J. Bernthal, & A. Byrd, 1990, *Journal of Speech and Hearing Disorders, 55,* 779–798.

TABLE 7–2. Age of acquisition (50% to 75% correct) of American English consonant clusters in word initial positions*.

Cluster	50%	75%	Cluster	50%	75%
tw	3;0	3;6	pr	4;0	6;0
kw	3;0	3;6	br	3;6	6;0
sp	3;6	5;0	tr	5;0	5;6
st	3;6	5;0	dr	4;0	6;0
sk	3;6	5;0	kr	4;0	5;6
sm	3;6	5;0	gr	4;6	6;0
sn	3;6	5;6	fr	3;6	6;0
sw	3;6	5;6	θr	5;0	7;0
sl	4;6	7;0	skw	3;6	7;0
pl	3;6	5;6	spl	5;0	7;0
bl	3;6	5;0	spr	5;0	8;0
kl	4;0	5;6	str	5;0	8;0
gl	3;6	4;6	skr	5;0	8;0
fl	3;6	5;6			

* = The Smit et al. data does not contain information for [ʃr] consonant clusters.

Complied from "The Iowa Articulation Norms Project and Its Nebraska Replication," by A. Smit, L. Hand, J. Frelinger, J. Bernthal, & A. Byrd, 1990, *Journal of Speech and Hearing Disorders, 55,* 779–798.

Idioms

Many children pronounce *yellow* with an initial [l] after they produce [j] correctly in a variety of different words and phonetic contexts. The initial [l], of course, results from an assimilation involving the [l] later in the word. Words that are pronounced much less accurately than other words in a child's vocabulary are called **regressive idioms**, while words that are pronounced much better than other words in a child's vocabulary are called **progressive idioms**. Idioms, both regressive and progressive, are usually excluded from consideration when performing an analysis of correct production of speech sounds, because most often such an analysis seeks to identify a child's typical way of speaking.

QUESTIONS

1. Which entire consonant classes are typically acquired by children before 3 years of age? (*Hint:* Use a 50% acquisition criterion for this and the following questions.)

2. Which fricative is typically acquired before 3 years of age?

3. Which classes of consonants are typically acquired after 3 years, 0 months and before 4 years, 6 months?

4. Which class of consonants is typically acquired at 4 years, 6 months of age?

5. Which class of consonant clusters is typically acquired at 3 years, 0 months of age? (*Hint:* Answers about consonant clusters require more description than did the answers about consonants.)

6. Which classes of consonant clusters are typically acquired after 3 years, 0 months of age and before 5 years, 0 months of age? (*Hint:* There is more than one way to describe these classes of consonant clusters, so your answer may differ somewhat from that in the back of the book.)

7. Which classes of consonant clusters are typically acquired at 5 years, 0 months of age?

8. Based on your answers, rank order the following words from earliest to latest in terms of which are likely to be pronounced correctly: *chew, spray, me, glue.*

Answer Sheet for Exercise 7–1: Consonants and Consonant Clusters

1. **Consonant classes:**

2. **Fricatives:**

3. **Consonant classes:**

4. **Consonant classes:**

5. **Consonant clusters:**

6. **Consonant clusters:**

7. **Consonant clusters:**

8. **Words:**

Exercise 7–2: Consonants and Consonant Clusters

This and the following exercise explore typical patterns and individual differences in the acquisition of consonants and consonant clusters. For reasons of space, the exercises only consider consonants and consonant clusters occurring in the beginning of words; the interested reader might perform similar analyses for sounds in other word and syllable positions.

SPEECH SAMPLES

See Appendix B.

QUESTIONS

1. By 2 years of age a child has mastered a number of word initial consonants. Place a check next to the word initial consonants on the accompanying table that the 4 children listed in Appendix B–1 through B–4 produced correctly in all words. Compare this to Smit et al.'s (1990) information for word initial consonants typically acquired before 3 years of age.

2. Answer the following questions about individual differences and typical patterns in consonant acquisition in children near 2 years of age.

   A. What is the range in number of acquired consonants?
   B. Compare the acquired consonant classes in Smit et al. (1990) to those of Amahl and Jake, the children whose acquisition of word initial consonants are least and most developed, respectively.
   C. Compare the children's acquisition of fricatives to each other and to Smit et al. (1990).

3. By 3 years, 6 months of age the "typical" child has acquired all the word initial English consonants, except for the interdental fricatives. Individual differences in consonant acquisition exist, however. The speech of a particular child may continue to contain errors. Rikki, although developing speech in a completely typical manner, has difficulty with a few word initial consonants (see Appendix B–6). Which consonants were they? (*Hint:* In Rikki's dialect the interdental fricatives are pronounced as alveolar stops.)

4. What is the sound class that includes both of Rikki's error sounds?

5. The speech of Taylor, a child 3 years, 6 months of age, contains an error in a word that begins with a liquid consonant (see Appendix B–8). What is the word?

6. Describe the error in question 5.

7. Taylor's error affects an individual sound, although at an earlier stage in development it may have been an error pattern that affected an entire sound class. What would this error be called if it were an error pattern?

8. By 5 years of age a child has typically acquired all the word initial English consonants, although random errors and errors in longer words with unfamiliar stress patterns may continue to occur. Max, a typically developing 5 year old child, has consistent difficulty pronouncing two word initial consonants (see Appendix B–10). Which consonants are they?

9. Describe Max's errors.

Answer Sheet for Exercise 7–2: Consonants and Consonant Clusters

1. **Word Initial Consonants at 2 Years of Age**

Sound	Smit et al., 1990	Hildegard	Kylie	Amahl	Jake
p					
t					
k					
b					
d					
g					
m					
n					
f					
θ					
s					
ʃ					
v					
ð					
z					
tʃ					
dʒ					
h					
j					
w					
l					
r					

2. A. **Smit et al.:**
   Hildegard:
   Kylie:
   Amahl:
   Jake:
   B. **Smit et al.:**
   Amahl:
   Jake:
   C. **Fricatives:**

3. **Consonants:**

4. **Sound class:**

5. **Word:**

6. **Description of error:**

7. **Error pattern:**

8. **Consonants:**

9. [s̬] =
   [r̥] =

Exercise 7–3: Consonants and Consonant Clusters

This exercise explores acquisition of consonant clusters in children from 2 to 5 years of age.

SPEECH SAMPLES

See Appendix B.

QUESTIONS

1. Many children do not produce any consonant clusters correctly at 2 years of age. Kylie and Jake are both exceptions to this general rule (see Appendix B–2 and B–4). Which word initial consonant clusters does each child produce correctly in all words?

2. Kylie and Jake's consonant clusters both begin with the same sound. Based on what you know about individual differences in articulation and phonological development, do you think that the first consonant clusters of all children begin with the same sound?

3. By 3 years, 6 months of age a child has typically mastered many but not all word initial consonant clusters. A child, for example, is expected to have acquired word initial [fl] consonant clusters, but is not expected to have acquired word initial [kl] and [kr] consonant clusters until approximately 4 years of age. To better see individual differences among typical patterns of acquisition, identify which of the children aged 3 years, 6 months old have acquired word initial [fl], [kl], and [kr] consonant clusters (see Appendix B–5 through B–8).

4. Describe typical patterns and individual differences in the acquisition of [fl], [kl], and [kr].

5. All the consonant clusters of English are typically acquired by 5 years of age, although, as always, individual differences in acquisition occur. The latest acquired consonant clusters typically are [θr], [spr], [spl], [str], and [skr]. Identify which of the children 5 years, 0 months of age have acquired [spr], [str], and [skr] (*Note:* [θr] and [str] do not often occur in the children's dialect).

6. Based on your answer to question five, describe typical patterns and individual differences in the acquisition of [spl], [sp], and [skr].

Answer Sheet for Exercise 7–3: Consonants and Consonant Clusters

1. **Kylie =**
   Jake =

2.

3. **Word Initial [fl], [kl], and [kr] Consonant Clusters**

Clusters	Smit et al., 1990	Rikki	Diane	Taylor	Tony
kl					
kr					
fl					

4.

5. **Word Initial [spl], [spr], and [skr] Consonant Clusters**

Clusters	Smit et al., 1990	Ryan	Shannon	Max	Puuala
spl					
spr					
skr		NT*			

* = not tested

6.

CHAPTER
8

Dialect

with Brian Goldstein

Dialect is a natural part of language, and dialect characteristics need to be identified in the speech of children in Stages 2 through 4 so that dialect patterns will not be mistaken for articulation and phonological disorders. Many dialects of English are spoken in the United States, including **African American English Vernacular (AAEV)**, **Hawaiian Island Creole (HC)**, and **Spanish-influenced English (SIE)**. The major dialect characteristics of AAEV, HC, and SIE are listed in Tables 8–1 through 8–3, respectively.

Local Norms, Community Values

Dialects vary by ethnic group, social class, region, city, and even neighborhood. The speech of an African American child in Seattle, for example, is not likely to contain the same dialect characteristics as an African American child living in Alabama. Further, a list of dialect characteristics does not offer insights into community values. For example, noting that persons using a certain dialect pronounce interdental fricatives as alveolar stops does not tell the clinician if the child's community either values or disvalues this characteristic of their dialect. The information in this section provides practice in identifying broad dialectal features in several ethnic groups. For all the reasons listed above, the information does not diminish the need for obtaining local norms and understanding community values.

TABLE 8–1. Major dialect patterns in African-American English Vernacular (AAEV).

Patterns	Examples
Stopping	
[θ] – [t]	*thought* is *tought*
[ð] – [d]	*this* is *dis*
Place changes between vowels and word finally	
[θ] – [f]	*bath* is *baf*
[ð] – [v]	*bathing* is *baving*
[ŋ] – [n]	*swing* is *swin*
Devoicing at ends of words	
[b] – [p]	*slab* is *slap*
[d] – [t]	*bed* is *bet*
[g] – [k]	*bug* is *buk*
Raising of [ɛ] before nasals	
[ɛ] – [ɪ]	*pen* is *pin*
Deletion	
V+ [r] – V + ∅	*more* is *mo*
CC# – C∅#	*nest* is *nes*
Vowel nasalization and nasal deletion	
V + N – nasalized vowel	*tame* is *tā*

Compiled from "Performance of Working Class African American Children on Three Tests of Articulation," by Cole & Taylor, 1990, *Language, Speech, and Hearing Serv-ices in Schools, 21,* 171–176.

TABLE 8–2. Major dialect patterns in Hawaiian Island Creole (HC).

Patterns	Examples
Stopping	
[θ] – [t]	*thick* is *tick*
[ð] – [d]	*this* is *dis*
Backing in environment of [r]	
[θr] – [tʃr]	*three* is *chree*
[tr] – [tʃr]	*tree* is *chree*
[str] – [ʃtr]	*street* is *shtreet*
Deletion	
V+ [r] – V + schwa	*here* is *hea*
CC# – C∅#	*nest* is *nes*

Compiled from "The Effects of Hawaiian Creole on Speech and Language Assessments," by D. Lyons, 1994, Unpublished master's project, Division of Speech Pathology and Audiology, University of Hawaii, Honolulu.

TABLE 8–3. Characteristics of Spanish-influenced English (SIE).

Patterns	Examples
Affrication	
/ʃ/ → [tʃ]	/fɪʃ/ → [fɪtʃ]
/j/ → [dʒ]	/jɛlo/ → [dʒɛlo]
Consonant Devoicing	
/z/ → [s]	/hɪz/ → [hɪs]
/dʒ/ → [tʃ]	/dʒɛl/ → [tʃɛl]
Nasal Velarization	
/n/ → [ŋ]	/fæn/ → [fæŋ]
Stopping	
/v/ → [b]	/ves/ → [bes]
/θ/ → [t]	/θat/ → [tat]
/ð/ → [d]	/ðo/ → [do]

Compiled from "Dialectal Variations," by A. Iglesias & N. Anderson, pp. 147–161. In J. Bernthal & N. Bankson (Eds.), 1993, *Articulation and phonological disorders*, (3rd ed.). New York: Prentice-Hall.

Exercise 8–1: Dialect

African American English Vernacular (AAEV) is spoken by many, but not all, African-Americans. AAEV shares many of linguistic features of "standard" American English, of other dialects of English (e.g., Southern English, Cockney English), and of other languages (Iglesias & Anderson, 1993). This exercise focuses on AAEV patterns in the speech of a child 7 years, 6 months of age (Goldstein, 1995).

SPEECH SAMPLE

Intended Words	Child
1. bathe	bev
2. pen	pɪn
3. house	haʊs
4. spoon	spū
5. skates	sket
6. stars	sta.əz
7. zipper	zɪpo
8. keys	kiz
9. that	dæt
10. shoe	ʃu
11. egg	ɛk
12. station	steʃʌ
13. fish	fɪʃ
14. sandwich	sæmwɪtʃ
15. thumb	θʌm

PROBLEM

Use Table 8–1 to help identify AAEV patterns in this child's speech. (**Hint:** Some words contain none or more than one AAEV pattern.) *The first word is an example and is answered for you.*

Answer Sheet for Exercise 8–1: Dialect

SPEECH SAMPLE

Intended Words	Child	AAEV Pattern(s)
1. bathe	bev	Place change
2. pen	pɪn	
3. house	haʊs	
4. spoon	spū	
5. skates	sket	
6. stars	sta.əz	
7. zipper	zɪpo	
8. keys	kiz	
9. that	dæt	
10. shoe	ʃu	
11. egg	ɛk	
12. station	steʃʌ	
13. fish	fɪʃ	
14. sandwich	sæmwɪtʃ	
15. thumb	θʌm	

Exercise 8–2: Dialect

Hawaiian Island Creole (HC), as its name suggests, is a dialect spoken by many persons in the Hawaiian Islands. HC tends to be spoken more often by those of Polynesian or Asian descent and by those living in rural areas. This exercise considers HC characteristics in the speech of Shannon, a typically developing child who is 5 years, 0 months of age.

SPEECH SAMPLE
See Appendix B–11.

QUESTIONS

1. Which words in Shannon's speech show the influence of the HC Stopping pattern?
2. What is the difference between Stopping as a dialect pattern and Stopping as an error pattern?
3. Which words in Shannon's speech show the influence of the HC pattern of Backing in the environment of [r]?
4. Backing affects [dr] consonant clusters in the speech of some HC speakers. Which of Shannon's words show this optional dialect pattern?
5. Why do you hypothesize Backing might occur in the environment of [r]? (**Hint:** Consider how [r] is produced.)
6. *For discussion:* Suppose a child speaks HC. She or he comes to you for an evaluation of a possible articulation and phonological disorder. You notice that the child Stops most fricatives, including those produced interdentally. Should you consider Stopping a dialect pattern or an error pattern?
7. *For discussion:* Should speech-language pathologists provide treatment to reduce dialect?

Answer Sheet for Exercise 8–2: Dialect

1. **Words:**

2. **Stopping:**

3. **HC pattern:**

4. **Words:**

5. **Hypothesis:**

6. *For discussion:*

7. *For discussion:*

Exercise 8–3: Dialect

Spanish-influenced English (SIE) is spoken by many persons whose families emigrated from Mexico, the Caribbean, and Spanish speaking Central and South America. This exercise provides an opportunity to analyze the speech of a boy 6 years, 0 months of age who speaks a variety of SIE (Gold-stein, 1995). Because SIE characteristics are better understood by those with some knowledge of Spanish, a capsule summary and an exercise on Spanish and its acquisition is provided in the appendix to this chapter.

Latino-Americans

Latino-Americans are the fastest-growing minority group in the United States. Currently, approximately 17 million Latinos reside in the United States, an increase of 2.3 million since the 1980 Census (Yates, 1988). Of that number, about 3 million are either in elementary or secondary schools and are thought to be either limited- or non-English speaking (U.S. Bureau of the Census, 1991). It is estimated that approximately 7% of those enrolled in school have some type of speech impairment (U.S. Bureau of the Census, 1991).

SPEECH SAMPLE

Intended Words	Child
1. van	bæn
2. beads	bits
3. cheese	tʃis
4. green	griŋ
5. yellow	dʒelo
6. feather	fedor
7. fish	fitʃ
8. glove	glʌb
9. ice cubes	aɪkjups
10. jump rope	tʃʌmrop
11. mouth	mat
12. Jason	dʒesoŋ
13. Santa Claus	santaklas
14. shoe	tʃu
15. spoon	spũŋ

PROBLEM

Use the information in Table 8–3 to identify SIE patterns in this child's speech. (**Hint:** Some words contain more than one SIE pattern.) *The first word is an example and is answered for you.*

Answer Sheet for Exercise 8–3: Dialect

Intended Words	Child	SIE Pattern(s)
1. van	bæn	Stopping
2. beads	bits	
3. cheese	tʃis	
4. green	griŋ	
5. yellow	dʒelo	
6. feather	fedor	
7. fish	fitʃ	
8. glove	glʌb	
9. ice cubes	aɪkjups	
10. jump rope	tʃʌmrop	
11. mouth	mat	
12. Jason	dʒesoŋ	
13. Santa Claus	santaklas	
14. shoe	tʃu	
15. spoon	spũŋ	

Exercise 8–4: Dialect

It is important to distinguish between dialect patterns and developmental errors in the speech of all children. This exercise provides an opportunity to identify dialect patterns and developmental errors in the speech of a child 6 years of age who speaks a variety of SIE (words adapted from Pollock & Keiser, 1990).

Why SIE?

Iglesias and Anderson (1993) outline four factors that may result in an individual's use of SIE. First, phones in English do not occur in Spanish. For example, [pʰ tʰ kʰ s v θ] occur in English but not in Spanish. Second, the distribution of consonants varies between the two languages. For example, only the consonants [s ɾ l n d] occur in word final position in Spanish. Third, differences in places of production of the same phonemes in the two languages. For example, /d/ in English is produced at the alveolar ridge compared to a dental place of production in Spanish. Fourth, for older Spanish-speakers acquiring English, the writing system may influence speech production. For example, the grapheme "z" is produced in English as both [s] as in *zoo* and as [ʒ] as in *azure*.

SPEECH SAMPLE

Intended Words	Child
1. pillow	pɪwo
2. toothache	tutek
3. feather	fɛdo
4. hello	xelo
5. football	tʊtbal
6. zebra	sibra
7. cowboy	taɪbɔɪ
8. office	apɪs
9. movie	mubi
10. book	bʊt

PROBLEM

Complete the following table, indicating which aspects of the child's speech result from SIE and which from developmental errors. Use Table 8–3 to identify SIE patterns, and indicate developmental errors using the x – y notation. *The first two words are examples and are answered for you.*

Answer Sheet for Exercise 8–4: Dialect

Intended Words	Child	SIE	Developmental
1. pillow	pɪwo		l – w
2. toothache	tutek	Stopping	
3. feather	fɛdo		
4. hello	xelo		
5. football	tʊtbal		
6. zebra	sibra		
7. cowboy	taɪbɔɪ		
8. office	apɪs		
9. movie	mubi		
10. book	bʊt		

APPENDIX

Standard Spanish

There are five primary vowels and 18 consonant phonemes in "standard" Spanish (Iglesias & Anderson, 1993). Although a "standard" version of Spanish is not actually spoken by anyone, describing a so-called standard form aids in the understanding of Spanish in general. The phonemes and allophones of Spanish are listed in Table 8–4.

Dialects

The two most prevalent dialects of Spanish in the United States are Southwestern United States (characterized by the Mexican-American dialect) and Caribbean (characterized by the Cuban and Puerto Rican dialects) (Iglesias & Anderson, 1993). Differing from English, in which dialectal variations are generally defined by vowel differences, Spanish dialectal changes primarily affect such large consonant classes as fricatives, liquids, glides, and nasals. Table 8–5 lists the primary dialect features of the Mexican, Cuban, and Puerto Rican forms of Spanish.

Acquisition of Spanish

Data on phonological development in normally developing Spanish-speaking children are described here and summarized in Table 8–6. Typically, by the time Spanish-speaking children who are developing normally reach the age of 3, they will use the dialect features of their community and will have mastered vowels and most consonants (e.g., Acevedo, 1991; De la Fuente, 1985; Fantini, 1985; Gonzalez, 1978; Mason, Smith & Hinshaw, 1976; Summers, 1982). By age 5, these children will only exhibit some difficulty with consonant clusters and certain phones, [x s ð ɲ r tʃ r l]. They will still, on occasion, exhibit Cluster Reduction, Syllable Deletion, deletion of stridents, and tap/trill /r/ deviation, but will likely have eliminated Fronting, Initial Consonant Deletion, Stopping, and Velar and Labial Assimilation (e.g., Bailey, 1982; Goldstein, 1988; Goldstein & Iglesias, in press; Gonzalez, 1978; Macy, 1979; Mason, Smith, & Hinshaw, 1976). In the early elementary school years, some Spanish-speaking children may show some, although intermittent, errors on the fricatives [x] and [s], the affricate [tʃ], the liquids [r r l], and consonant clusters (e.g., Gonzalez, 1978; Mason, Smith, & Hinshaw, 1976).

TABLE 8–4. Phonemes and allophones of "Standard" Spanish.

Phonemes (/ /) and Allophones ([ ])					
Vowels					
Close /i/ /u/		*Mid* /e/ /o/		*Open* /a/	
[i] [u]		[e] [o]		[a]	
Consonants					
Oral stops /p/ /t/ /k/		/b/	/d/	/g/	
[p] [t] [k]		[b β v]	[d ð]	[g ɣ]	
Nasal stops /m/	/n/	/ɲ/			
[m]	[n ŋ]	[ɲ]			
Fricatives and affricate	/f/	/s/	/x/	/tʃ/	
	[f ɸ]	[s ʰ ø]	[x h]	[tʃ]	
Liquids /l/ /ɾ/ /r/					
[l] [ɾ l i] [r R x]					
Glides /w/ /j/					
[w u gw] [j i dʒ]					

TABLE 8–5. Characteristics of Spanish dialects.

Patterns	Examples	Dialects
Stops		
/b/ → [v]	/boka/ → [voka] *mouth*	M
/d/ → ∅	/sed/ → [se] *thirsty*	C
/k g/ → ∅	/doktoɾ/ → /doktoɾ/ *doctor*	M
/n/ → [ŋ]	/xamon/ → [hamoŋ] *ham*	C PR
Fricatives		
/f/ → [ɸ]	/kafe/ → [kaɸe] *coffee*	PR
/s/ → ∅	/dos/ → [do] *two*	M C PR
/s/ → ʰ	/dos/ → [doʰ] *two*	M C PR
/ð/ → ∅	/dedo/ → [deo] *finger*	M C PR
/x/ → [h]	/xamon/ → [hamon] *ham*	M C PR
Liquids		
/ɾ/ (tap) → ∅, CC	/koɾta/ → [kotta] *to cut*	C
/ɾ/ → [l]	/koɾtaɾ/ → [koltaɾ] *to cut*	PR (C rare)
/ɾ/ → [i]	/koɾtaɾ/ → [koitaɾ] *to cut*	PR (rural)
/r/ (trill) → [R]/[x]	/pero/ → [peRo]/[pexo] *dog*	PR (M rare)

Key: M = Mexican; C = Cuban; PR = Puerto Rican

TABLE 8–6. Major milestones in the acquisition of Spanish.

Acquisition at Age 3
- Mastery* of vowels
- Consonants *not* typically mastered include [g f s ɲ ɾ r] and consonant clusters

Acquisition at Age 5
- Mastery of most consonants
- Intermittent errors on [ð x s ɲ tʃ ɾ r l] and consonant clusters
- Occasionally will exhibit Cluster Reduction, Syllable Deletion, Stridency Deletion, and deviations on tap/trill /r/
- Typically have suppressed Fronting, Initial Consonant Deletion, Stopping, Velar and Labial Assimilation

Acquisition at Age 7
- Infrequent errors on fricatives [x] and [s], affricate [tʃ], liquids [ɾ r l] and consonant clusters

* = Mastery defined as 90% accurate.

Exercise 8–5: Dialect

A complete evaluation of a Spanish-speaking child includes an analysis of the child's speech in his or her native language. This exercise provides an opportunity to analyze the speech of a 7-year-old child in her native Spanish (Goldstein, 1995).

SPEECH SAMPLE

Intended Words	Child
1. boka	oka
2. xaβon	haβon
3. floɾ	foɾ
4. dos	dot

(continued)

SPEECH SAMPLE *(cont'd)*

Intended Words	Child
5. deðo	eðo
6. maɾtijo	mattijo
7. gato	gago
8. xuɣo	kuɣo
9. kasa	kata
10. bloke	boke
11. weβo	welo
12. tɾen	tɾem

PROBLEM

Use the information in Tables 8–4 through 8–6 to distinguish Spanish dialect characteristics from likely and unlikely developmental errors in the speech of this child (for detailed discussion of Spanish and its development see Goldstein & Iglesias, in press). *The first two words are examples and are answered for you.*

Answer Sheet for Exercise 8–5: Dialect

Intended Words	Child	Likely	Unlikely	Dialect	English
1. boka	oka		✓		mouth
2. xaβon	haβon			✓	soap
3. floɾ	foɾ				flower
4. dos	dot				two
5. deðo	eðo				finger
6. maɾtijo	mattijo				hammer
7. gato	gago				cat
8. xuɣo	kuɣo				juice
9. kasa	kata				house
10. bloke	boke				block
11. weβo	welo				egg
12. tɾen	tɾem				train

CHAPTER
9

Acquisition Strategies

nalysis of acquisition strategies is undertaken with children in Stage 2 and early Stage 3. **Acquisition strategies** represent approaches to learning how to speak. The existence of acquisition strategies serves to remind us that children are actively engaged in the process of articulation and phonological development. The hallmarks of various acquisition strategies are listed in Table 9–1.

REGRESSIONS

Regressions are temporary losses of articulation and phonological abilities lasting from a day to months. Some regressions involve a loss in phonetic accuracy in a single word, and others may alter previously "correct" stress patterns, syllable shapes, or sound classes (Bleile & Tomblin, 1991; Menn, 1976). Regres-

TABLE 9–1. Major articulation and phonological acquisition strategies.

Strategies	Hallmark
Regressions	The client temporarily loses a speech ability. A temporary regression may last from days to months.
Favorite sounds	The client uses a sound (sometimes an unusual one, such as syllabic [s]) in place of many other sounds.
Selectivity	The client "picks and chooses" words that contain sounds and sound sequences that he or she already produces.
Word recipes	The client's words are organized into only a few sound patterns.
Homonyms	The client either avoids or seeks words that are pronounced as homonyms.
Word-based learning	The client's pronunciation of a sound varies, depending on the word in which it occurs.
Gestalt learning	The client knows "the tune before the words."

sions appear to arise as a child generalizes and overgeneralizes regular ways to say words. Similar to morphological overgeneralization (e.g., when a preschooler overgeneralizes the past tense marker to say, *I goed home*), articulation and phonological regressions actually represent progress in development.

FAVORITE SOUNDS

Favorite sounds are consonants and vowels that occur with unusually high frequency in a child's speech. A favorite sound, for example, might be an [s] that a child uses to pronounce all words that in adult language begin with fricatives, stops, or affricates (Ferguson & Macken, 1983). Although having favorite sounds is not a disability, extensive use of favorite sounds may result in increased numbers of homonyms and may signify difficulty in acquiring a repertoire of diverse speech sounds.

SELECTIVITY

Selectivity is the ability of some children to "pick and choose" the sounds and sound sequences they will attempt to pronounce. In general, children appear to choose words that contain sounds already in their expressive vocabularies (Schwartz, 1988; Schwartz & Leonard, 1982). A child, for example, may have an expressive vocabulary containing words beginning with [t] and [k] and only be willing to attempt to pronounce new words that begin with the same sounds.

WORD RECIPES

Word recipes are simple formulas that some children appear to use to simplify the task of speaking. The term word recipes is intended to convey that some children, like some inexperienced cooks, use a very few recipes over and over again (Menn, 1976; Waterson, 1971). A child, for example, might have two word recipes that he or she uses to pronounce almost all words. One word recipe might be, "All words that are monosyllables in the adult language are pronounced as CV and the consonant is [d]," and the other word recipe might be, "All words that are multisyllabic in the adult language are pronounced CVCV and both consonants are identical in place of production." Children whose acquisition strategies include word recipes may find it easier to acquire words that follow their word recipes. More

negatively, the speech of children who follow this strategy is often highly unintelligible, because these children only have a few means to pronounce a large number of sounds and syllables.

HOMONYMS

Homonyms are words that sound alike but have different meanings. Some children appear unbothered by the number of homonyms in their speech; others appear to produce unusual pronunciations to avoid having too many homonyms (Ingram, 1975). Children who appear to tolerate a great many homonyms are called **homonym seeking**, and children who appear to avoid homonym are called **homonym avoiding**. A child's degree of homonym is determined simply by dividing the number of different homonyms in the child's expressive vocabulary by the total number of words.

WORD-BASED LEARNING

Word-based learning employs words to organize the articulation and phonological systems. The distinguishing trait of word-based learning is that a child's pronounciation of a sound is dependent on the word in which it occurs (Ferguson & Farwell, 1975). For example, a word-initial [p] in the adult language may be pronounced by the child as [b] in one word, as [t] in another word, and as [p] or [s] in other words. Word-based learning disappears as a child discovers regular ways to say words, which typically occurs as the child's expressive vocabulary grows to 50 or more words. The change from word-based learning to rule-based learning may be one source of articulation and phonological regressions. To illustrate, the child in the above example might generalize [t] to all words that begin with [p] in the adult language, resulting in a temporary regression in words that previously had been pronounced with an initial [p]. Although word-based learning is not a form of disability, persistent use of this acquisition strategy results in extensive variability in the production of sounds.

GESTALT LEARNING

Gestalt learning typically involves "learning the tune before the words" (Peters, 1977, 1983). Children prone to gestalt learning may accurately produce sentence intonation (the tune), although the pronunciation of words within the sentence may be poor. Sometimes children who pronounce the intonation of sentences better than the sounds in the sentence are said to be speaking "jargon." Children speaking "jargon" are often extremely difficult to understand, because the sounds within the words are highly inaccurate.

A Small Revolution

A small revolution in the study of articulation and phonological development occurred from the mid-1970s to the mid-1980s. Before then, models of articulation and phonological development tended to view children as relatively passive learners. Linguistic models defined acquisition as the unfolding of a genetically controlled program of development, and models in speech-language pathology viewed acquisition as the gradual lessening of motoric limitations through a combination of physical development and motor practice. The revolution that began in the mid-1970s was to view children as active constructors of their articulation and phonological systems. Delineation of acquisition strategies, in attempting to identify the resources children bring to the challenge of learning how to talk, remains an important legacy of that fertile decade of research.

Exercise 9–1: Acquisition Strategies

This exercise asks you to match a description to the appropriate acquisition strategy.

QUESTIONS

1. How a child says a sound depends on the word in which it occurs.

2. The child produces the intonation of a sentence, although the sounds within the sentence are highly inaccurate.

3. The child produces a sound more accurately at an earlier age than at a later age.

4. The child appears to seek words that sound alike.

5. The child appears to avoid words that sound alike.

6. The child has only a few ways to pronounce words.

7. The child seems to pick and choose the sounds he or she will say.

Answer Sheet for Exercise 9–1: Acquisition Strategies

1. **Strategy:**

2. **Strategy:**

3. **Strategy:**

4. **Strategy:**

5. **Strategy:**

6. **Strategy:**

7. **Strategy:**

Exercise 9–2: Acquisition Strategies

One of the first exercises in this section analyzed the phonetic inventory of Leslie, a child 11 months of age whose entire intelligible vocabulary consisted of 4 words. The article in which Leslie was profiled created a considerable stir in academic circles when it was first published—not so much for Leslie's phonetic inventory, but for the restricted nature of the words Leslie attempted to pronounce (Ferguson, Peizer, & Weeks, 1973). If you cover Leslie's pronunciations with your hand and look only at the intended words on the left, a striking finding emerges: the words Leslie attempts are all similar in their stress, syllables, and sounds. Although it might be sup-posed that Leslie's parents only taught their daughter words with certain articulation and phonological characteristics, the authors of the original study thought otherwise, and subsequent research has borne them out. In fact, what Ferguson and his colleagues hypothesized was that Leslie selected the words she pronounced based on the stress, syllables, and sounds they contained. A decade later, research confirmed that selectivity was a fairly common acquisition strategy among children under 20 months of age. The present exercise provides an opportunity to reanalyze the original case of selectivity.

What Do Children Select?

In a series of clever experiments Schwartz and his colleagues have shown that a child selects words that contain stress patterns, syllables, and sounds that the child already produces (Schwartz, 1988; Schwartz & Leonard, 1982). A child, for example, whose expressive vocabulary contains words beginning with [m] is more likely to choose to pronounce new words beginning with that sound. Selectivity may be one important source of individual differences between children. To illustrate, a child whose first word is *mommy* may select more words with one set of stress, syllable, and sound patterns, while a child whose first word is *bird* may select words with very different articulation and phonological characteristics. For the purposes of clinical care, selectivity is important because it suggests that clients in early Stage 2 may more readily acquire words containing articulation and phonological characteristics of words already in their spoken vocabulary.

SPEECH SAMPLE

Intended Words	Leslie
1. daddy	dædæ
2. mommy	mama
3. doggie	gaga
4. patty (cake)	bæbæ

QUESTIONS

1. What do the words Leslie attempted have in common in terms of stress patterns? (*Hint:* For this exercise, analyze the words Leslie attempted rather than Leslie's pronunciations.)

2. What do the words Leslie attempted have in common in terms of sequence of syllables?

3. The consonants in the words Leslie attempted are restricted in their place of production. What places of production occur?

4. The consonants in the words Leslie attempted are also restricted in their manner of production. What manners of production occur?

5. What vowel or vowels do all the words Leslie attempted share in common?

Answer Sheet for Exercise 9–2: Acquisition Strategies

1. **Stress patterns:**

2. **Sequence of syllables:**

3. **Place of production:**

4. **Manner of production:**

5. **Vowels:**

Exercise 9–3: Acquisition Strategies

Some cooks make many different dishes that all end up tasting like spaghetti. Some children do the same thing to words, reducing the vast phonetic complexity of speech to a few word recipes (Menn, 1976). Waterson (1971) was one of the first investigators to describe this phenomenon. This exercise offers you the opportunity to analyze information from Waterson's study of a child approximately 1 year, 6 months of age.

SPEECH SAMPLE

Intended Words	Child
1. fish	ɪʃ~
	ʊʃ
2. brush	bɪʃ
3. window	ɲeɲe
4. fetch	ɪʃ
5. another	ɲaɲa
6. dish	dɪʃ
7. finger	ɲeɲe~
	ɲiɲi
8. Randell	ɲaɲe
9. vest	ʊʃ

QUESTIONS

1. Describe the first consonant in the third word in terms of place, manner, and voicing. (**Hint:** This exercise only considers the child's productions. If needed, cover the intended words with your hand.)

2. The words in the list contain two word recipes. Consider the child's pronunciations and then indicate by word number which words belong in each recipe.

3. A "trick" in analyzing word recipes is to determine which articulation and phonological characteristics all the words in a recipe share in common. What stress pattern is shared by all the words in the word recipe that includes *fish*?

4. Does the word recipe that includes *fish* share a common sequence of syllables? If yes, what is it?

5. Does the word recipe that includes *fish* share common consonants and vowels? If yes, what are they?

6. Does the word recipe that includes *fish* share common distinctive features for consonants and vowels? If yes, what are they?

7. Based on your answers above, describe the word recipe for the words that include *fish*. (**Hint:** Summarize the common articulation and phonological characteristics you discovered above.)

8. Perform a similar analysis for the word recipe that contains *window* as you did for the word recipe that contained *fish*.

9. Based on your answers above, describe the word recipe for the words that include *window*. (**Hint:** As with the other word recipe, summarize the common articulation and phonological characteristics you discovered above.)

Answer Sheet for Exercise 9–3: Acquisition Strategies

1. **Distinctive features:**

2. **First recipe:**
   Second recipe:

3. **Stress pattern:**

4. **Syllables:**

5. **Consonants and vowels:**

6. **Distinctive features:**

7. **Word recipe:**

8. A. **Stress:**
   B. **Sequence of syllables:**
   C. **Consonants:**
   D. **Vowels:**
   E. **Consonant distinctive features:**
   F. **Vowel distinctive features:**

9. **Word recipe:**

Exercise 9–4: Acquisition Strategies

Regressions in speech development have been recognized and discussed since at least the 1940s, when a German linguist named Leopold described how his daughter's pronunciation of *pretty* regressed in phonetic accuracy over a period of many months (Leopold, 1947). It was not until the mid 1970s, however, that investigators came to fully appreciate that sound classes as well as individual words could regress in development. This exercise allows you to analyze a famous case of regression in a child from between one year, 6 months to 1 year, 8 months of age (Menn, 1976).

SPEECH SAMPLE

Age	Jacob	
	kaka*	cracker/cookie
Before 1;6:27	[kaká]	[káka] or [kúki]
1;6:27	kaká	
1;7:10		kʌkí
1;7:17	gak	
1;7:24	káka	kʌkí
1;7:27	káka~ káka	kʌkí
1;8:18		kúki
1;8:22	gʌ́ga~ kʌ́ka	

* = *Kaka* [kaká] is a Greek word learned from a babysitter that means feces.

QUESTIONS

1. Which syllable in *kaka* receives primary stress before 1;6:27?

2. When does the regression in *kaka* occur?

3. Describe the regression in *kaka* in your own words.

4. Which syllable in *cracker* and *cookie* receives primary stress before 1;6:27?

5. When does the regression in *cracker* and *cookie* begin and end?

6. Describe the regression in *cracker* and *cookie* in your own words.

7. Suppose you taught Jacob the word *cackle* on 1;7:24. If your hypothesis about the regression that affects *cracker* and *cookie* is correct, how would Jacob pronounce the stress pattern in *cackle*?

8. Jacob's regression in the pronunciation of *cracker* and *cookie* is difficult to explain as a physical problem in producing primary stress on the first syllable. Why?

9. *For discussion:* What is your hypothesis for why Jacob changes the stress patterns in *kaka*, *cracker*, and *cookie*?

Answer Sheet for Exercise 9–4: Acquisition Strategies

1. **Primary stress:**

2. **Date:**

3. **Description:**

4. **Primary stress:**

5. **Dates:**

6. **Regression:**

7. *Cackle***:**

8. **Explanation:**

9. *For discussion:*

SECTION
III

Analysis of Articulation and Phonological Disorders

OVERVIEW

The chapters in this section address issues in assessment. As in the previous section, the long period over which articulation and phonological development occurs is divided into 4 broad stages. For convenience, these stages are summarized again in Table III–1.

TABLE III–1. Primary characteristics of four stages in articulation and phonological development.

Stages	Age Range in Typically Developing Children	Primary Characteristics
Stage 1	0–12 ms	Vocalizations seldom if ever used for referential purposes
Stage 2	12–24 ms	Small expressive vocabulary (less than 100 words)
Stage 3	2–5 yrs	Errors affecting sound classes
Stage 4	5 yrs and older	Errors affecting late-acquired consonants, consonant clusters, and unstressed syllables in more difficult multisyllabic words

Steps in the Assessment

An articulation and phonological assessment consists of three steps. The first step is the **initial observation** during which the clinician listens to the client's spontaneous speech, making a few notes about particular speech errors and formulating an initial impression about the client's level of intelligibility. Approximately 3 to 5 minutes are allotted for the initial observation. The second step is **collection of the speech sample** for later analysis using either standardized instruments, nonstandardized measures, or a combination of both. Approximately 10 to 30 minutes are allotted for the collection of the speech sample. The third step is **hypothesis testing**, which is undertaken to gather additional information about the client's articulation and phonological disorder. For example, hypothesis testing might determine if a client's production of *key* as [ti] during the collection of the speech sample was an isolated error or the result of an error pattern. Hypothesis testing typically requires from a few minutes to 30 minutes, depending on the nature and complexity of the client's articulation and phonological disorder.

CHAPTER
10

Measures of Severity and Intelligibility

easures of severity and intelligibility are typically used to determine eligibility for treatment.

SEVERITY

Severity is the degree of a client's articulation and phonological disorder. A primary use of measures of severity is to determine treatment eligibility. The most frequently used severity assessment tools are clinical judgment scales. Percentage of development offers yet another option to assess severity. Less often used, but more theoretically and methodologically rigorous means to measure severity are percentage of consonants correct (PCC) and the articulation competence index (ACI). The ACI is a new measure used to calculate the percentage of distortions in a client's speech (Shriberg, 1993). However, the ACI is not calculated in this book, because the speech samples were not obtained following the procedures appropriate to that instrument.

Clinical Judgment Scales of Severity

While clinical judgment scales are useful with clients in all stages, their greatest use is with clients in Stages 3 and 4 in situations in which a quick means to assess large numbers of potential clients is needed. **Clinical judgment scales** are based on the judgment of one or more speech-language clinicians familiar with the client who are asked to rank the client's articulation and phonological development compared to persons of similar age or level of cognitive development. Two examples of clinical judgment scales of severity are provided in Table 10–1.

Percentage of Development

Percentage of development is used with clients in all levels of articulation and phonological development. **Percentage of development** is the difference between a client's chronological age and the age equivalent corresponding to his or her level of articulation and phonological development. A child 3

TABLE 10–1. Two clinical judgment scales of severity.

Type	Categories
4-Point Scale	1 = No disorder
	2 = Mild disorder
	3 = Moderate disorder
	4 = Severe disorder
3-Factor Scale	A = The client's speech has or in the future is likely to have an adverse affect on his or her social development and educational progress.
	B = The client's speech calls attention to itself.
	C = The client's speech is delayed relative to developmental age norms.

years of age, for example, whose articulation and phonological development approximated a child 2 years of age would have a delay of 33%. States differ in the specific cutoff criteria they use to establish the need for articulation and phonological treatment.

Percentage of Consonants Correct (PCC)

The PCC is used with clients whose speech contains multiple substitutions and deletions; most typically, these clients are in Stage 3. As its name suggests, the **PCC** measures severity as a function of the percentage of consonants the client produces correctly out of the total number of consonants the client attempts (Shriberg & Kwiatkowski, 1982). Scoring instructions for the PCC are provided in the appendix of this chapter.

INTELLIGIBILITY

Intelligibility is the factor most frequently cited by both speech-language clinicians and laypersons in

deciding the severity of a client's articulation and phonological disorder (Gordon-Brannan, 1994; Shriberg & Kwiatkowski, 1983). Importantly, **intelligibility** is sometimes also used as a criterion to select targets for treatment. Three means used to assess intelligibility are **clinical judgment scales of intelligibility**, **frequency of occurrence**, and **effects of error patterns on intelligibility**.

Clinical Judgment Scales of Intelligibility

Judgment scales of intelligibility are used with clients in Stages 2 through 4; like severity scales, intelligibility scales are most useful within clinical settings where clinicians can perform large numbers of assessments to identify clients in need of treatment. As with severity judgment scales, a judge or judges (typically, speech-language clinicians) familiar with the client are asked to rank the client's speech compared to persons of similar chronological or developmental age. Examples of two types of clinical judgment scales of intelligibility are contained in Table 10–2.

Why Isn't Intelligibility Used More Often?

As the major purpose of speaking is to be understood, why isn't intelligibility used more often in determining eligibility for services and in treatment target selection? The answer is that, interestingly enough, the correlation between intelligibility and the number of consonants pronounced correctly is relatively low (r = .42) (Shriberg & Kwiatkowski, 1982, 1983). Some nonspeech factors thought to have an important influence on intelligibility include the listener's familiarity with the speaker and the topic and the nature of the social environment in which the speech occurs.

Frequency of Occurrence

A frequency of occurrence analysis is used with clients in Stages 2 through 4. Frequency of occurrence is the relative frequency of sounds in the language of the client's community. **Frequency of occurrence** is related to intelligibility based on the hypothesis that—all other matters being equal—the higher a sound's relative frequency of occurrence, the greater the sound's impact on intelligibility. The relative frequency of English consonants is listed in Table 10–3.

TABLE 10–2. Two clinical judgment scales of intelligibility.

Type	Categories
3-Point Scale	1 = Readily intelligible
	2 = Intelligible if topic is known
	3 = Unintelligible, even with careful listening
5-Point Scale	1 = Completely intelligible
	2 = Mostly intelligible
	3 = Somewhat intelligible
	4 = Mostly unintelligible
	5 = Completely unintelligible

TABLE 10–3. Relative frequency of occurrence of English consonants.

Consonant		Rank	Percentage	Consonant		Rank	Percentage
t	____	1	13.7	p	____	13	3.9
n	____	2	11.7	b	____	14	3.5
s	____	3	7.1	z	____	15	3.0
k	____	4	6.0	ŋ	____	16	2.5
d	____	5	5.8	f	____	17	2.4
m	____	6	5.6	j	____	18	2.2
l	____	7	5.6	ʃ	____	19	1.5
r	____	8	5.2	v	____	20	1.2
w	____	9	4.8	θ	____	21	0.9
h	____	10	4.2	tʃ	____	22	0.7
ð	____	11	4.1	dʒ	____	23	0.6
g	____	12	4.1	ʒ	____	24	0.0

Compiled from "Computer-Assisted Natural Process Analysis (NPA): Recent Issues and Data," by L. Shriberg and J. Kwiatkowski, 1983, in J. Locke (Ed.) *Seminars in Speech and Language, 4*, 397.

Error Patterns

Assessment of the effects of error patterns on intelligibility is typically undertaken with clients in Stage 3 to help select short-term goals. Although clinicians have long speculated about the effects of **error patterns** on intelligibility (Hodson, 1986), the relationship between error patterns and intelligibility has only recently begun to be studied (Leinonen-Davies, 1988; Yavas & Lamprecht, 1988). Results from Leinonen-Davies (1988) indicate that Fronting had the most effect on intelligibility in word-initial position, followed by Gliding, Prevocalic Voicing, Stopping, and Cluster Reduction. Final Consonant Deletion affects intelligibility most severely in word-final position, followed by Fronting and Word Final Devoicing.

Exercise 10–1: Measures of Severity and Intelligibility

Measures of severity provide a means to help make decisions about treatment eligibility. This exercise offers an opportunity to determine severity of involvement using severity judgment scales, PCC, and percentage of development. The exercise is based on the speech of E, a child who is 2 years, 8 months of age, and whose utterances all are single words (Bleile, Stark, & Silverman McGowan, 1993). E was born prematurely. She received a tracheosto-my when she was approximately 3 months of age subsequent to bronchopulmonary dysplasia (BPD), a lung problem sometimes resulting from medical efforts to save children with immature lungs too weak to reliably provide the breaths of life. E's tracheostomy was removed when she was 2 years, 4 months of age, approximately 4 months before the following words were spoken.

Spontaneous or Elicited Speech?

Spontaneous speech is the preferred sampling technique because it is most representative of how a client talks (Ingram, 1994; Morrison & Shriberg, 1992; Morrison & Shriberg, 1994). The major limitation of obtaining spontaneous speech samples is the length of time it can take to transcribe them, especially if the client speaks in sentences of three or more words. Further, longer utterances usually must be tape recorded for transcription, which adds greatly to the time needed to complete an analysis. For this reason, many clinicians prefer to spend a few minutes early in the assessment session listening to the client's spontaneous speech, perhaps making notes about particular speech errors and the client's level of severity and/or intelligibility. The initial impression of the client's spontaneous speech is then used to guide the subsequent analysis of the client's elicited speech.

E at 6 Years Old

E is 6 years of age and is doing well in a regular first grade classroom. E's mother reports that E's speech is understood by all, but that she receives speech services 20 minutes a week for problems involving a lateral lisp and several consonant clusters.

SPEECH SAMPLE

Intended Words	E
1. daddy	dædə
2. hi	haɪ
3. down	da
4. mom	mɑm
5. hop	bɑp
6. water	wɑwa
7. book	bʊk
8. bow	boʊ
9. baby	bʌbə
10. up	ʌp
11. please	baɪ
12. bye	baɪ
13. bag	baɪ
14. bubble	bʌ
15. pop	bɑp
16. ball	bɔ
17. Pop Pop*	pɑp pɑp

* = Pop Pop is the family name for grandfather.

QUESTIONS

1. Suppose three clinicians familiar with E select to measure severity using use a 4-point clinical judgment scale such as that depicted in Table 10–1. What severity ranking would E receive if the scores of three clinicians are 2, 3, and 3, respectively? (**Hint:** First, calculate E's severity score, then round the results to the nearest whole number, and then assign a severity rating.)

2. Instead of a 4-point scale, suppose the clinicians selected a 3-factor clinical judgment scale similar to that shown in Table 10–1. What severity ranking would E receive if the clinician's scores were 2, 2, and 3? (*Hint:* This measure does not assign a rating using a mild-to-severe scale, so your answer will be a numerical score such as 1.2, 3.0, etc.)

3. Suppose a clinician decided to measure severity using the PCC rather than a clinical judgment scale. Read the instructions for calculating PCC in the appendix of this chapter. Next, answer the following questions.

   A. How many consonants does E attempt and how many does she produce correctly? (*Hint:* Count the number of consonants E attempts and the number she produces correctly. To illustrate, *daddy* contains two consonants, both of which E produces correctly, yielding a score of 2/2 for that word.)

   B. What is E's PCC score? What is her severity rating?

4. Percentage of development offers another option for determining severity of involvement. Suppose a clinician selects this option and determines that E's articulation and phonological development approximates that of a child 15 months of age based on the number and type of consonants in her word initial and word final consonant inventory. What is E's percentage of development? (*Hint:* You will need to convert E's chronological age into months.)

5. *For discussion:* Compare and contrast the merits and limitations of clinical judgment scales, the PCC, and percentage of development.

6. *For discussion:* What do you consider the merits and limitations of severity as a method to establish treatment eligibility?

Answer Sheet for Exercise 10–1: Measures of Severity and Intelligibility

1. **Severity score:**

2. **Severity score:**

3. A. **Attempted:**
      Correct:
   B. **PCC:**

4.

5. *For discussion:*

6. *For discussion:*

Exercise 10–2: Measures of Severity and Intelligibility

This exercise provides an opportunity to become more familiar with the simple calculations and somewhat more complex ideas that underlie the use of intelligibility measures. Three concepts of intelligibility are considered: clinical judgment scales, frequency of occurrence of consonants, and effects of error patterns. The exercise is based on the speech of Dora, a child who is 2 years, 9 months of age and whose hearing and language abilities are within normal limits.

SPEECH SAMPLE

See Appendix C–1.

QUESTIONS

1. As with clinical judgment scales of severity, clinical judgment scales of intelligibility are used to determine if a person is eligible for treatment. Two commonly encountered intelligibility scales are shown in Table 10–2. Use Table 10–2 to answer the following questions.

   A. Suppose three clinicians score Dora's speech as 1, 1, and 2 on a 3-point clinical judgment scale of intelligibility. What is Dora's intelligibility rating?

   B. Suppose the three clinicians had decided to use a 5-point scale instead. The scores they gave Dora's speech were 3, 4, and 4. What is Dora's intelligibility rating?

2. The frequency of occurrence of a sound is sometimes used in conjunction with factors such as developmental age norms and better abilities to select treatment targets. For this question, however, use frequency of occurrence as the sole criterion for treatment target selection.

   A. Dora has difficulty pronouncing both word initial [s] and [z]. Which consonant is a more likely treatment target with intelligibility as a criterion? Why?

   B. Dora has difficulty pronouncing all the word initial voiceless fricatives. Which voiceless fricative is the most likely treatment target with intelligibility as a criterion? Why?

   C. Dora has difficulty pronouncing both [k] and [l] in word initial position. Which consonant is a more likely treatment target with intelligibility as a criterion? Why?

3. The effects of various error patterns on intelligibility offers a relatively new method for selecting error patterns for remediation. As with the exercises on relative frequency of sounds, answer the following questions using the effects of error patterns on intelligibility as the sole criterion in selecting treatment targets.

   A. Dora's speech contains both Fronting and Stopping in word initial position. Which error pattern is the more likely focus of treatment, if an intelligibility criterion is used? Why?

   B. Suppose you decide to provide treatment to overcome Fronting. Use the information in Table 10–3 to select which sound should receive remediation, [k] or [g]. Why?

   C. Dora's speech contains both Final Consonant Deletion and Fronting in word final position. Why do you suppose that Final Consonant Deletion has a greater effect on intelligibility than Fronting?

4. *For discussion:* What are the merits and limitations of clinical judgment scales in establishing eligibility for treatment?

5. *For discussion:* What are the merits and limitations of relative frequency of sounds and the effects of error patterns on intelligibility as methods for selecting treatment targets?

Answer Sheet for Exercise 10–2: Measures of Severity and Intelligibility

1. A. **Intelligibility score:**
   B. **Intelligibility score:**

2. A. **Treatment target:**
   B. **Treatment target:**
   C. **Treatment target:**

3. A. **Error pattern:**
   B. **Error pattern:**
   C. **Error pattern:**

4. *For discussion:*

5. *For discussion:*

APPENDIX

Percentage of Consonants Correct (PCC)

A. Instructions

Calculate the client's PCC using the procedures described below and on the following pages. The level of severity needed to obtain articulation and phonological services varies by clinical setting; a score of 50–65% or less is recommended for most client populations, and a less stringent criterion—65% or higher—is recommended for clients at risk for future articulation and phonological difficulties.

B. Step 1: Collect Data and Identify Utterances

The following data collection procedures are used:

- Obtain a continuous speech sample of between 50 and 100 utterances.
- Determine the meaning of the utterances.
- Identify any dialect characteristics (example: *aks* or *ask* in AAEV).
- Identify casual speech pronunciations (example: *Cheat yet?* for *Did you eat yet?*).
- Identify allophones (example: [ɾ] for [t] in *butter*).

C. Step 2: Determine Exclusion Criteria

The following data are excluded from analysis:

- All unintelligible and partially intelligible utterances.
- Vowels (including [ɚ]).
- The addition of consonants in front of vowels (example: *hit* for *it*) because the target is a vowel.
- Consonants in the third or more repetition of the same word, if the pronunciation does not change (example: count only the first two instances of [b] in three or more repetitions of *bee* [bi bi bi]).
- Beyond the second consonant in successive utterances with the same pronunciation, but score all consonants if the pronunciation changes.

D. Step 3: Identify Errors in the Remaining Data

Follow these criteria to identify consonant errors:

- Score dialect, casual speech, and allophones based on the consonant the client intended (example: *aks* for *ask* is correct in AAEV, but *ats* is incorrect).
- Score a consonant as incorrect if in doubt about whether it is correct or incorrect.
- Score consonant deletions as incorrect (example: *be* for *bed*).
- Score consonant substitutions as incorrect (example: *bee* for *pea*).
- Score partial voicing of initial consonants as incorrect.
- Score distortions (no matter how mild) as incorrect.
- Score additions of a sound to consonant as incorrect (example: *mits* for *miss*).
- Score initial [h] and [n/ŋ] substitutions in stressed syllables as incorrect, but not in unstressed syllables (example: *swin* for *swing* is incorrect, but *jumpin* for *jumping* is correct).

E. Step 4: Calculate PCC

Perform the following calculation to determine PCC:

1. Formula

$$\frac{\text{total number of correct consonants}}{\text{total number of intended consonants}} \times 100 = \text{PCC}$$

2. Example

$$\frac{70 \text{ consonants correct}}{100 \text{ consonants attempted}} \times 100 = 70\%$$

F. Step 5: Determine Level of Severity

Indicate the client's level of severity using the following scale:

85% or higher	=	Developing typically	_____
65% to 85%	=	Mild to moderate disorder	_____
50% to 65%	=	Moderate to severe disorder	_____
<50%	=	Severe disorder	_____

CHAPTER
11

Developmental Age Norms

Developmental age norms list the average ages at which children typically acquire articulation and phonological behaviors. Developmental age norms are used both to select treatment targets and to establish the age corresponding to a client's articulation and phonological development. For example, a child 4 years of age whose major articulation and phonological abilities corresponded to those of a child 2 years of age would likely be assessed as having approximately the articulation and phonological skills of a child 2 years of age. In certain treatment approaches, articulation and phonological behaviors that a client is most delayed in acquiring would be selected as early treatment targets (see Chapter 15). The areas of development for which age norms are most frequently obtained in clinical settings are phonetic inventories, error patterns, and consonants and consonant clusters. For convenience, the information on these topics presented in the beginning of Section 2 is repeated here with slight modifications.

Delay Versus Disorder?

Developmental age norms provide a useful way to compare a person's articulation and phonological development to his or her age mates. Some investigators place so great an emphasis on this comparison that they prefer the term delay to disorder. I prefer the term disorder because I do not typically make clinical decisions based solely on the extent to which a person is delayed relative to his or her age mates. To illustrate, if a person were teased because of speech, I might accept the individual into treatment, even if the person's delay in articulation and phonological development was only slight. Further, if the speech development of a 4-year-old child approximated that of a 2-year-old, I might recommend language stimulation rather than articulation and phonological treatment, if the child's other cognitive and developmental skills also approximated that of a 2-year-old.

PHONETIC INVENTORIES

Analysis of **phonetic inventories** is performed with clients in Stage 2 and early Stage 3, when clients are still relatively restricted in their speech abilities. The analysis describes a client's ability to pronounce distinctive features, sounds, syllables, and stress patterns. The analysis does not specify whether or not clients speak "correctly." A phonetic inventory analysis, for example, might indicate a client's consonant inventory contains [t], [k], and [s], but would not indicate whether [t] was produced for [t] in *two* or for [z] in *zebra*.

Developmental age norms exist for phonetic inventories of consonants. Consonant inventories based only on children's intelligible utterances are presented in Table 11–1 (Stoel-Gammon, 1985), and consonant inventories based both on intelligible and unintelligible utterances are presented in Table 11–2 (Robb & Bleile, 1994). The information in Table 11–2 is based on an experimental study (n = 7) and, consequently, should be used with some caution. The developmental level of a client's consonant inventory is that most closely approximating the number and type of the client's established consonants. For an analysis restricted only to intelligible words, a consonant is considered established when it occurs in at least two different words (the criteria used in the original studies). For an analysis of both intelligible and unintelligible words, a consonant is considered established when it occurs in at least three different words (the criteria used in the original study).

ERROR PATTERNS

An error pattern analysis is performed with clients in Stage 2 and 3. The analysis describes a client's

TABLE 11–1. Typical consonant inventories in children 15 through 29 months of age based on analysis of intelligible utterances.

Age	Position	Number of Consonants	Typical Consonants
15 mos*	Initial	3	b d h
	Final	none	—
18 mos*	Initial	6	b d m n h w
	Final	1	t
24 mos*	Initial	11	b d g t k m n h w f s
	Final	6	p t k n r s
29 mos**	Final	14	b d g p t k m n h w j f s l
	Final	11	d p t k m n ŋ f s ʃ tʃ

* = Compiled from "Phonetic Inventories, 15–24 Months: A Longitudinal Study," by C. Stoel-Gammon, 1985, *Journal of Speech and Hearing Research, 28,* 505–512.

** = Compiled from "Phonetic Inventories of 2- and 3-Year-Old Children," by A. Dyson, 1988, *Journal of Speech and Hearing Disorders, 53,* 89–93.

TABLE 11–2. Typical consonant inventories in children 12 through 24 months of age based on analysis of intelligible and unintelligible utterances.

Age	Position	Number of Consonants	Typical Consonants
12 mos	Initial	5	b d g m h
	Final	1	m
18 mos	Initial	6	b d m n h w
	Final	2	t s
24 mos	Initial	10	b d p t k m n h s w
	Final	4	t k n s

Compiled from "Consonant Inventories of Young Children From 8 to 25 Months," by M. Robb and K. Bleile, 1994, *Journal of Clinical Linguistics and Phonetics, 8,* 295–320.

speech errors affecting sound classes. **Error patterns** encompass both what are traditionally called phonological processes and certain types of articulation errors. The term error pattern is used in this book to avoid biasing the discussion toward either an articulation or phonological perspective. The appendix at the end of Chapter 6 contains definitions of 23 common and uncommon error patterns. Of 12 common error patterns, Stoel-Gammon and Dunn (1985) identify 7 that disappear by 3 years of age (Prevocalic Voicing, Velar Assimilation, Labial Assimilation, Reduplication, Final Consonant Deletion, Fronting, and Syllable Deletion), and 5 error patterns that typically disappear after 3 years of age (Epenthesis, Gliding, Cluster Reduction, Final Consonant Devoicing, and Stopping).

Clinical care often requires knowing how often an error pattern occurred compared to the total number of times it might have occurred. One possible use of this information is to help select short-term treatment goals (see Chapter 14). To illustrate, many clinicians find treatment success occurs more readily if the short-term goal is an error pattern that affects some, but not all of the words it might affect. Another possible reason to determine the frequency with which an error pattern occurs is to establish how often an error pattern occurs before treatment. For example, a pretest might indicate that an error pattern occurred 60% of the time and a posttest might indicate that the same error pattern now occurs 30% of the time. A simple means to categorize error patterns by their frequency of occurrence is provided in Table 11–3.

CONSONANTS AND CONSONANT CLUSTERS

Analysis of **consonants and consonant clusters** is undertaken with clients in Stages 2 through 4. The analysis describes a client's ability to pronounce individual consonants and consonant clusters. The ages at which consonants and consonant clusters are typically acquired are listed in Tables 11–4 and

TABLE 11–3. Percentage and whole number criteria for disappearance of error patterns.

Categories	Percentages	Whole Numbers* (5 Chances)	Whole Numbers* (10 Chances)
Highly frequent	75 to 100	4/5–5/5	8/10–10/10
Frequent	50 to 74	3/5	5/10–7/10
Present	25 to 49	2/5	3/10–4/10
Disappearing	1 to 24	1/5	1/10–2/10
Disappeared	0	0/5	0/10

* = Whole numbers refer to the number of different words. For example, 3/5 means the error pattern occurred in three of five words.

TABLE 11–4. Age of acquisition (50% to 75% correct) of American English consonants averaged across both word initial and word final positions.

Consonant	50%	75%	Consonant	50%	70%
m	<3;0	<3;0	f	<3;0	3;6
n	<3;0	<3;0	v	3;6	4;6
ŋ	<3;0	7;6*	θ	4;6	6;0
h	<3;0	<3;0	ð	4;6	5;6
w	<3;0	<3;0	s	3;6	5;0
j	<3;0	3;6	z	4;0	6;0
p	<3;0	<3;0	ʃ	3;6	5;0
t	<3;0	<3;0	tʃ	3;6	6;0
k	<3;0	<3;0	dʒ	3;6	4;6
b	<3;0	<3;0	r	3;6	6;0
d	<3;0	<3;0	l	3;6	6;0
g	<3;0	<3;0			

* = Transcriber difficulties may have resulted in this sound being listed as acquired at 7:6.

Compiled from "The Iowa Articulation Norms Project and Its Nebraska Replication" by A. Smit, L. Hand, J. Frelinger, J. Bernthal, & A. Byrd, 1990, *Journal of Speech and Hearing Disorders, 55,* 779–798.

11–5 (Smit, Hand, Frelinger, Bernthal, & Byrd, 1990). To be considered acquired, a sound met two criteria: (1) at least 50% of both males and females correctly produced the sound in word initial and word final positions (consonants) or word initial position (consonant clusters), and (2) the percentage of subjects correctly producing the sound at subsequent age levels never dropped below 50%. Lastly, clinical care requires a means to identify the percentage of times a client can produce a sound. A simple means to determine this percentage is provided in Table 11–6.

TABLE 11–5. Age of acquisition (50% to 75% correct) of American English consonants clusters in word initial positions*.

Cluster	50%	75%	Cluster	50%	70%
tw	3;0	3;6	pr	4;0	6;0
kw	3;0	3;6	br	3;6	6;0
sp	3;6	5;0	tr	5;0	5;6
st	3;6	5;0	dr	4;0	6;0
sk	3;6	5;0	kr	4;0	5;6
sm	3;6	5;0	gr	4;6	6;0
sn	3;6	5;6	fr	3;6	6;0
sw	3;6	5;6	θr	5;0	7;0
sl	4;6	7;0	skw	3;6	7;0
pl	3;6	5;6	spl	5;0	7;0
bl	3;6	5;0	spr	5;0	8;0
kl	4;0	5;6	str	5;0	8;0
gl	3;6	4;6	skr	5;0	8;0
fl	3;6	5;6			

* = The Smit et al. data does not contain information for [ʃr] consonant clusters.

Compiled from "The Iowa Articulation Norms Project and Its Nebraska Replication" by A. Smit, L. Hand, J. Frelinger, J. Bernthal, & A. Byrd, 1990, *Journal of Speech and Hearing Disorders, 55,* 779–798.

TABLE 11–6. Percentage and whole number criteria for acquisition of consonants and consonant clusters.

Categories	Percentages	Whole Numbers* (5 Chances)	Whole Numbers* (10 Chances)
Mastered	75 to 100	4/5–5/5	8/10–10/10
Acquired	50 to 74	3/5	5/10–7/10
Emerging	10 to 49	2/5	1/10–4/10
Rare	1 to 10	0/5	1/10
Absent	0	0/5	0/10

* = Whole numbers refer to the number of different words. For example, 4/5 means the sound was produced correctly in 4 of 5 words.

Exercise 11–1: Developmental Age Norms

A phonetic inventory analysis is often used both to help select words for a client's expressive vocabulary as well as to establish the age equivalency that most closely corresponds to a client's articulation and phon-ological development. This exercise is based on the speech of Johnny, a boy with Down syndrome whose entire expressive vocabulary at 3 years, 11 months of age consists of 8 words (Bleile, 1995).

Johnny

Johnny is a friendly, rambunctious child of 6 years. After nearly 2 years of therapy, Johnny's expressive vocabulary consists of many hundreds of words. Johnny typically speaks in short two- to four-word sentences composed mainly of vowels, stops, glides, and a few fricatives. His intelligibility is good to familiar listeners when the sentences are short and the topics are known.

SPEECH SAMPLE

Intended Words	Johnny
1. bubble	bʌ
2. baby	bʌ
3. pig	pɪ
4. dog	gɔ
5. go	gɔ
6. pop	gɔ
7. in	gɔ
8. moo	gɔ

QUESTIONS

1. Which word initial consonants occur in two or more words? (*Hint:* For this and the following questions, do not consider the intended words. If necessary, review the pertinent exercises in Chapters 1 and 2.)

2. Which word final consonants occur in two or more words?

3. Which distinctive features do all of Johnny's word initial consonants share in common?

4. How do [b] and [g] differ from each other in terms of distinctive feature(s)?

5. Compare your analysis of Johnny's consonant inventory to the information in Table 11–1. Which age most closely approximates Johnny's consonant inventory?

6. Suppose Johnny is a child who is selective in the words he will attempt to pronounce (see Chapter 9). Based on your analysis, which word do you hypothesize that Johnny will most likely attempt: *pie, bug,* or *toe*?

Answer Sheet for Exercise 11–1: Developmental Age Norms

1. **Word initial consonants:**

2. **Word final consonants:**

3. **Common distinctive features:**

4. **Different distinctive features:**

5. **Age equivalence:**

6. **Words:**

Exercise 11–2: Developmental Age Norms

This exercise offers the opportunity to perform an analysis on the speech of a client with a somewhat more developed phonetic inventory than that of the child in the previous exercise. The speech on which this exercise is based comes from a 2-year, 3-month-old child named Matt (Carpenter, 1995). Matt's development appears completely typical except in the area of articulation and phonology.

SPEECH SAMPLE

Intended Words	Matt
1. mama	mama
2. ball	ba
3. eyes	aɪ
4. bear	bɝ ~ bɛr
5. bye bye	baɪbaɪ~ bʌbʌ
6. dog	dɑ
7. cake	geɪ
8. yeah	jæ
9. bus	bʌ
10. all	aʊ
11. kitty	gigi
12. mine	maɪ
13. Babette	bæbə
14. Kate	keɪkeɪkeɪ
15. moo	mun
16. wow	waʊ
17. apple	ʔæʔæ
18. duck	duʔ~ dʌk
19. up	ʌ
20. yes	ɛs

QUESTIONS

1. Which word initial consonants occur in two or more words?

2. Which word final consonants occur in two or more words?

3. Compare your results to the information in Table 11–1. Which age most closely approximates Matt's consonant inventory? Briefly describe the rationale for your choice of a particular age equivalency. (**Hint:** Remember that age norms are just averages. You should not expect Matt's consonant inventory to be exactly the same as the normative information.)

4. The criterion you select to determine when a sound or syllable is acquired can have an important influence on your analysis. This and the previous exercise used occurrence in two words to determine if a consonant was acquired. The two-word criterion was selected so that you could compare your results to normative information. To better understand the difference a change in criterion can make, identify Matt's consonant inventory using a one-word, two-word, and three-word acquisition criterion.

5. *For discussion:* Each criterion results in a different analysis of Matt's consonant inventory. Which criterion do you believe best represents Matt's consonant inventory?

Answer Sheet for Exercise 11–2: Developmental Age Norms

1. **Word initial:**

2. **Word final:**

3. **Age equivalence:**

4.

Matt's Consonant Inventory

Criterion	Inventory	
	Word Initial	Word Final
1-word		
2-word		
3-word		

5. *For discussion:*

Exercise 11–3: Developmental Age Norms

As in the previous exercises, in this exercise you are asked to analyze a client's consonant inventory and to compare your results to developmental age norms. For this exercise, however, the developmental age norms are for both intelligible and unintelligible words. The client whose speech forms the basis of the present exercise is a 20-month-old child named Ethan (Lee, 1994). Ethan was born 2 months prematurely through induced labor because, as Ethan's mother reports, "the fetus had stopped growing in utero."

SPEECH SAMPLE

Intended Words	Ethan
1. balloon	bʌwʊ
2. banana	bʌ
3. bus	bʌ
4. duck	dæ
5. dog	gɔ
6. down	dʌm
7. cake	te
8. car	dʌ
9. cookie	tuʔi
10. kite	haɪ
11. sock	tʌ
12. sun	tʌ
13. nose	noʊ
14. eat	di
15. apple	ʌbʌ
16. up	ʌb
17. in	ʌɸ
18. ?	əgʌ
19. ?	ʌm
20. ?	hʌhoʊ
21. ?	hʌm
22. ?	tɪbʊ
23. ?	kʌhoʊ
24. ?	gʌʔ
25. ?	nʌ
26. ?	gæ
27. ?	tʌ
28. ?	gʌdɪ
29. ?	hæm
30. ?	tɪ

QUESTIONS

1. What consonants occur in word initial position? (*Hint:* A consonant must occur in three or more words to be included in Ethan's phonetic inventory, as that criterion was used in the study that provides the normative information.)

2. Which consonants occur in word final position?

3. Which developmental age most closely approximates Ethan's consonant inventory according to the information in Table 11–2?

Answer Sheet for Exercise 11–3: Developmental Age Norms

1. **Word initial:**

2. **Word final:**

3. **Age equivalence:**

Exercise 11–4: Developmental Age Norms

Similar error patterns occur in the speech of persons both with and without articulation and phonological disorders. The challenge of analyzing the speech of persons with articulation and phonological disorders lies in shaping the information from the evaluation to develop a treatment plan. The present exercise indicates how the evaluation of error patterns is used as a rationale for treatment and to help select treatment targets. This exercise is based on the speech of a child named Tess (see Appendix C–2 for the complete speech sample). Tess is 4 years, 4 months of age, bilingual (English and Korean), and is reported to be mildly delayed in the development of both languages. Tess's mother reports a normal prenatal and birth history, but that Tess did not say her first words until 2 years of age. Tess is an only child and lives in an extended family household in which Korean is the primary language. Tess' exposure to English is primarily through her preschool. An audiological evaluation indicates hearing within normal limits.

Word Probes

Many times it is necessary to determine the frequency with which an error pattern occurs. However, this procedure often is time consuming, especially if the clinician is attempting to count a number of different error patterns in a relatively long list of words. (To see this, try counting the number of possible occurrences of Stopping in a word list in Appendix C that contains over 50 words.) An alternative procedure is to use the initial speech sample to help identify error patterns that are likely short-term goals and then obtain short (5- to 10-word) word probes to determine how frequently specific error patterns occur. This procedure takes a few minutes in most cases and is useful both in selecting short-term goals and in serving as a treatment pretest.

SPEECH SAMPLE

Intended Words	Tess
4. popcorn	pɑtə
10. cannot	tænə
11. cat	tæ~
	tæt
12. coffee	tɑpi
13. cookie	tʊti
14. Cookie Monster	tuti mɑntə
15. cow	taʊ
16. crab	dəwæb~
	tu.æ
17. clown	taʊn
22. because	bitɑ
28. broken	bɔti.ɛn
29. doctor	doktə
34. grandma	dænəmɑ~
	dæmɑ
50. sticker	tɪtə
52. skate	peɪt
53. chicken	tɪtɛm
61. homework	hɔmwʊ̃
70. look	jut
75. okay	oʊteɪ

QUESTIONS

1. Which error pattern most frequently affects Tess' pronunciation of [k] and [g]? Give an example of a word that is affected by this error pattern. (*Hint:* This exercise does not contain any patterns affecting [k] and [g] that are the result of the influence of Korean.)

2. Based on your answer to the first question, show that Tess may be delayed in articulation and phonological development.

3. Tess' speech also evidences Stopping. Use developmental age norms as the criterion to decide whether Fronting or Stopping should be the primary treatment focus. (*Hint:* For this question ignore the possibility of treating both error patterns.)

4. Suppose (based on the speech sample in Appendix C–2) you as Tess' clinician are fairly certain that Fronting is a good short-term treatment goal for Tess. What five words could you use as evaluation tools and for a possible pretest to determine the frequency of occurrence of Fronting in word initial and word final positions? (*Hint:* Think of word probes as very flexible tools. For this example, test for Fronting in word initial and final position. Depending on the error patterns in a client's speech, however, a word probe might be restricted to a single word position or expanded to include more sounds.)

5. Suppose that the results of your word probe indicate that Fronting occurs in two of five words. Categorize Fronting according to the system shown in Table 11–3.

Answer Sheet for Exercise 11–4: Developmental Age Norms

1. **Error pattern:**
   Example:

2.

3.

4. **Possible words:**

5. **Category:**

Exercise 11–5: Developmental Age Norms

This exercise provides another opportunity to perform an error pattern analysis in conjunction with developmental age norms. The exercise is based on the speech of a 2 years, 9 month old child named Dora (see Appendix C–1 for the complete speech sample). Dora's history is unremarkable except for having an older brother receiving services for speech problems. Dora's hearing and language abilities are within normal limits.

A Few Words About Percentages

A table of percentages gives the impression that articulation and phonological analysis requires a great deal of computation. However, most clinicians are far too busy to make extensive computations feasible. Instead of exact numbers, think of percentages as providing general guidelines. To illustrate, **highly frequent** error patterns occur with few or no exceptions, while **disappearing** error patterns still occur, but have many, many exceptions. Similarly, a **mastered** consonant or consonant cluster is produced correctly on all or nearly all occasions, while a **rare** consonant or consonant cluster is produced correctly on occasion, but rarely.

SPEECH SAMPLE

Intended Words	Dora
4. telephone	bæbən
5. tricycle	taɪtɪtoʊ
14. bananas	nænəz
18. bus	bʌş
21. blocks	bwaʃ
23. give	dɪb
26. monster	mɑnsə
30. fishing	pɪʃɪn
31. feathers	pɛɾəs
32. fits	bɪts
33. find	faɪn
34. scissors	tɪzɔz
35. sun	tʌn
36. soap	soʊp
37. socks	ʃɑʃ
38. stop	tɑp
39. sleeping	pipɪn
40. shovel	şʌbl̩
44. zoo	su
45. zipper	ti
56. leaf	wif
61. ice cream	aɪtim

QUESTIONS

1. What error pattern affects Dora's pronunciation of fricatives?

2. Is this error pattern expected to occur in the speech of children of Dora's age? (**Hint:** The word list does not contain dialect patterns.)

3. This and the following questions allow you to compare two procedures in calculating percentage of occurrence of error patterns. What is the percentage of occurrence of Stopping in Dora's speech based on the word list in the answer sheet? (**Hint:** *Telephone* provides an example of how to fill in the table.)

4. Categorize Stopping according to the system shown in Table 11–3.

5. Dora's clinician undertook several short word probes. Determine the percentage of occurrence of Stopping in the word probe on the answer sheet.

6. Categorize Stopping according to the system shown in Table 11–3.

7. *For discussion:* What do you see as the merits and limitations of the two approaches to determining frequency of occurrence of error patterns?

Answer Sheet for Exercise 11–5: Developmental Age Norms

1. **Error pattern:**

2.

3.

Calculation of Percentage of Occurrence

Words	Dora	Stopping
4. telephone	bæbən	1/1
5. tricycle	taɪtɪtoʊ	
14. bananas	nænəz	
18. bus	bʌṣ	
21. blocks	bwɑʃ	
23. give	dɪb	
26. monster	mɑnsə	
30. fishing	pɪʃɪn	
31. feathers	pɛɾəs	
32. fits	bɪts	
33. find	faɪn	
34. scissors	tɪzɔz	
35. sun	tʌn	
36. soap	soʊp	
37. socks	ʃɑʃ	
38. stop	tɑp	
39. sleeping	pipɪn	
40. shovel	ṣʌbl̩	
44. zoo	su	
45. zipper	ti	
56. leaf	wif	
61. ice cream	aɪtim	
Total:		/
Percentage:		

4. **Category:**

5.

Word Probe

Words	Dora	Stopping
1. sun	tʌn	1/1
2. fun	pʌn	
3. bus	bʌs	
4. zoo	ṣu	
5. maze	meɪz	
Total:		/
Percentage:		

6. **Category:**

7. *For discussion:*

Exercise 11–6: Developmental Age Norms

Developmental age norms for consonants and consonant clusters serve several important purposes. For example, the presence of errors on sounds typically acquired below the client's developmental or chronological age is often used to justify treatment. Further, within many clinical approaches, treatment is more likely to focus first on earlier developing sounds than on those typically produced correctly at later ages. The present exercise offers the opportunity to analyze the consonants and consonant clusters in the speech of a child 6 years, 8 months of age whose name is Billy (Wolfe, 1994). Billy was referred to the clinic for problems with "r." Billy's medical, developmental, and social history are unremarkable. Billy's hearing was tested and was found to be within normal limits and he scored at the 94th percentile in receptive vocabulary on the *Peabody Picture Vocabulary Test-Revised* (Dunn & Dunn, 1981). The word list that follows was obtained during the initial evaluation and contains Billy's pronunciation of [r] in various word positions (see Appendix C-8 for the complete speech sample).

SPEECH SAMPLE

Intended Words	Billy
5. car	kɑr
6. cream	krim
7. cry	kwaɪ
11. brush	bʌʃ
13. drum	dr̥ʌm
15. green	gwin
16. great	gr̥ɛt
30. ring	r̥ɪŋ
31. rabbit	r̥æbət

QUESTIONS

1. At what age is [r] acquired in nonclusters by 50% of children? By 75% of children?

2. Explain how the information from the first question indicates that Billy may be delayed in articulation and phonological development.

3. Billy's ability to pronounce [r] in several consonant clusters was also assessed. Identify the consonant clusters that were assessed and the 50% and 75% developmental age norms for these sound combinations.

4. Explain how the information from the third question indicates that Billy may be delayed in articulation and phonological development.

5. After completing the initial evaluation, Billy's clinician decided that she wanted more information about [r] in nonclusters in word initial position, because she considered that a likely treatment target. Calculate Billy's percentage of errors on [r] using the word probe on the answer sheet. *The calculation of* rain *is an example and has been answered for you.*

6. Categorize [r] according to the system shown in Table 11–6.

Answer Sheet for Exercise 11–6: Developmental Age Norms

1. **[r]:**

2.

3.

Developmental Age Norms for Consonant Clusters

Consonant Clusters	Developmental Age Norms	
	50%	75%
kr		
br		
dr		
gr		

4.

5.

Word Probe

Words	Billy	Correct
1. rain	reɪn	1/1
2. row	woʊ	
3. run	ɾʌn	
4. root	rut	
12. row	woʊ	
15. ring	ɾɪŋ	
17. ray	ɾeɪ	
Total:		/
Percentage:		

6. **Category:**

Exercise 11–7: Developmental Age Norms

This exercise provides an opportunity to perform a consonant and consonant cluster analysis of a client in late Stage 3 of articulation and phonological development. The client whose speech is the basis of this exercise is named Dee. Dee is a child 7 years, 5 months of age who has received intermittent speech-language therapy since she was 3 years of age. Dee's medical and developmental history are unremarkable.

SPEECH SAMPLE

See Appendix C–9.

QUESTIONS

1. Which word initial consonants does Dee pronounce correctly? Which consonants does Dee pronounce incorrectly? (*Hint:* To be considered correct, a consonant must be produced correctly in all instances. Be sure to exclude from consideration all pronunciations resulting from possible dialect influence. Because Dee spoke a variety of Hawaiian Island Creole, the possible dialect patterns to exclude include [tʃ] and [dʒ] for [t] and [d], respectively, when followed by [r], and [t] and [d] for the voiceless and voiced interdental fricative, respectively.)

2. Perform the same analysis for word final consonants, indicating which consonants are and are not pronounced correctly. (*Hint:* Ignore consonants that occur in consonant clusters, and exclude [l] and [r] if they are pronounced as schwa, which is a pattern in Hawaiian Island Creole.)

3. Perform the same analysis for word initial consonant clusters, indicating which consonant clusters are and are not pronounced correctly.

4. Use the information from the first three questions to argue that Dee may be delayed in articulation and phonological development. (*Hint:* A simple way to make this argument is to focus your discussion on the sounds that Dee produces incorrectly.)

5. Dee pronounces word initial [j] incorrectly in *yellow*, most likely as the result of assimilation to [l]. Develop a word probe of three words to determine if Dee typically pronounces word initial [j] as [l].

6. Only a selection of consonant clusters was evaluated during the initial evaluation. Develop a word probe containing three words to determine how Dee pronounces [sp] word initial consonant clusters.

Answer Sheet for Exercise 11–7: Developmental Age Norms

1. **Correct:**
   Incorrect:

2. **Correct:**
   Incorrect:

3. **Correct:**
   Incorrect:

4.

5. **Word probe:**

6. **Word probe:**

CHAPTER
12

Better Abilities

When analyzing a client's speech, it is equally (or more) important to determine the client's areas of strength as it is to establish the client's deficit areas. The analysis of **better abilities** is undertaken to identify the client's more advanced articulation and phonological skills. The results of these analyses often are used to help select treatment targets. The primary types of analyses of better abilities are stimulability, key environments, key words, and phonetic placement and shaping.

Why Assess Better Abilities?

The purpose of analyses of better abilities is to determine if a client has some capacity to pronounce potential treatment targets. To illustrate, the speech sample might indicate a client pronounces [s] as [t]. An analysis of better abilities is undertaken to discover if the client is able to pronounce this sound during imitation (**stimulability testing**), in specific words (**key words**), in special phonetic contexts (**key environments**), or in response to direct instruction (**phonetic placement and shaping**). Although analysis of better abilities does not guarantee treatment success, most (but not all) clinicians believe that treatment proceeds more swiftly and the client is less frustrated if at the start of the treatment the client demonstrates some capacity to produce the treatment target.

STIMULABILITY TESTING

Stimulability testing is performed routinely with clients in Stages 2 through 4. **Stimulability** is the ability to say a treatment target correctly during delayed or immediate imitation. A client who pronounces [k] correctly during imitation, for example, is considered stimulable for [k]. The logic behind stimulability testing is that sounds that can be produced correctly during imitation are easier for clients to acquire than treatment targets that cannot be imitated.

KEY ENVIRONMENTS

Analysis of key environments is performed with clients from Stage 2 through Stage 4. A **key environment** is a phonetic environment in which the client is able to successfully produce a sound or class of sounds. Key environments often are syllable and word positions, but may also be the presence of other sounds. An example of a word (and syllable) key environment is a client who is only able to produce velar stops at the ends of words. Although individual differences in key environments are extensive, the following is a list of "first bets" as to the phonetic contexts in which to look for key environments:

- The beginning of words is the most common key environment for most consonants.
- Between vowels is sometimes a key environment for voiced consonants, especially voiced fricatives.
- The end of syllables and words is sometimes a key environment for voiceless consonants.
- The end of syllables and words is sometimes a key environment for velar consonants. Another key environment for velar stops may be before back vowels in the same syllable, as in *go*.
- The beginning of syllables and words before a front vowel is sometimes a key environment for alveolar consonants, as in "tea."

KEY WORDS

Analysis of key words is performed with clients from Stage 2 through Stage 4. **Key words** occur when a client's success in producing a sound is limited to a few specific words. Many times key words are of special importance to the client. Names of favorite friends and characters in television series are "first bets" when trying to find key words. Key words, however, need not be "special" to the client, and, in fact, any word can be a key word.

PHONETIC PLACEMENT AND SHAPING

Brief trials using phonetic placement and shaping techniques are performed with more mature and cognitively advanced clients in Stage 3 and clients in Stage 4. **Phonetic placement and shaping techniques** physically direct a client to produce a sound. A phonetic placement technique for [t], for example, might involve directing the client to touch his or her tongue tip to the alveolar ridge. A shaping technique for [t] might help a client shape [t] from [d].

Exercise 12–1: Better Abilities

Better abilities represent flexible options rather than exclusive choices. The existence of multiple methods to assess better abilities is our recognition that no single technique is appropriate for all clients. This exercise focuses primarily on stimulability testing and phonetic placement and shaping techniques, two widely used analyses of better abilities. The client whose speech forms the basis of this exercise is a 5-year, 2-month-old female child named Stacy (see Appendix C–4 for the complete speech sample). Stacy's medical, social, and developmental history are unremarkable. The results of speech-language evaluation indicates that Stacy's sole area of deficit lies in articulation and phonological development.

Assessing Better Abilities

The analysis of better abilities typically begins with consideration of a speech sample. After the sample is collected, the clinician scans down the transcription, looking for possible key words and key environments to test using word probes. If the client is willing and able to imitate, the clinician may ask him or her to imitate the words in the speech sample that contain articulation and phonological errors. Alternately, if the client's speech contains a great number of errors, the clinician may only ask him or her to imitate those errors that are likely treatment targets. Lastly, depending on the client's level of cognitive development, the clinician may attempt to help the client pronounce potential treatment targets using simple phonetic placement and shaping techniques. The entire time required to perform an analysis of better abilities typically ranges from a few minutes to 15 minutes.

SPEECH SAMPLE

Intended Words	Stacy	Stimulability Testing
2. Power Rangers	paʊwʊweɪndəs	
5. toothbrush	tubwəs	tubwəʃ
30. brush	bwʌs	
37. matches	mæsɪz	mæsɪz
42. fish	fɪs	fɪʃ
47. sandwich	sæwɪs	
54. shoe	su	ʃu
57. chair	sɛr	sɛr
58. jars	zɑz	zɑz
64. witch	wɪs	wɪs
72. orange	ɔɪns	
73. angels	ænzʊs	

QUESTIONS

1. What is the name of the error pattern that affects Stacy's pronunciation of postalveolar fricatives and affricate?

2. One way to perform stimulability testing is to ask the client to imitate a selection of words pronounced incorrectly during the initial speech sample. The results of such an approach is depicted on the right side of the speech sample. Describe the results of this analysis.

3. Another option (not necessarily the preferred one in many situations, since it requires more time to perform) is to develop a word probe for the client to imitate. Develop a six-word word probe that tests each of the affected consonants in word initial and word final position. (*Hint:* The voiced postalveolar fricative is not tested in this example because that sound occurs in few English words.)

4. Suppose Stacy had not been stimulable for [ʃ]. While procedures for performing phonetic placement and shaping techniques are available, developing your own techniques helps to better understand the principles on which they are built. For this reason, develop a simple phonetic placement technique for [ʃ] (*Hint:* Spend a moment thinking about how [ʃ] is produced, and then develop simple instructions to teach the sound.)

5. Develop a simple shaping technique to develop [ʃ] from [s]. (*Hint:* Spend a moment thinking about the difference between alveolar and postalveolar fricatives and then develop a simple set of instructions to guide the client from producing a voiceless alveolar fricative to producing a voiceless fricative in the postalveolar position.)

6. *For discussion:* What do you consider the merits and limitations of stimulability testing?

7. *For discussion:* What do you consider the strengths and limitations of phonetic placement and shaping techniques?

Answer Sheet for Exercise 12–1: Better Abilities

1. **Error pattern:**

2. **Words:**

3. **Stimulability results:**

4. **Key environments or key words:**

5. **Shaping:**

6. *For discussion:*

7. *For discussion:*

Exercise 12–2: Better Abilities

Analysis of key words and key environments can be undertaken in clients from Stage 2 through Stage 4. The previous exercise focused on the speech of a client in late Stage 3; the present exercise considers key words and key environments in the speech of a client in Stage 2. The client, identified as E, was born prematurely, and received a tracheostomy when she was approximately 3 months of age subsequent to bronchopulmonary dysplasia (BPD), a lung problem sometimes resulting from medical efforts to save children whose immature lungs are too weak to provide the breaths of life (Bleile, Stark, & Silverman McGowan, 1993). E's tracheostomy tube was removed when she was 2 years, 4 months of age. The following words were spoken 4 months after this decannulation and were E's entire expressive vocabulary at that time.

SPEECH SAMPLE

Intended Words	E
1. daddy	dædə
2. hi	haɪ
3. down	da
4. mom	mɑm
5. hop	bɑp
6. water	wɑwa
7. book	bʊk
8. bow	boʊ
9. baby	bʌbʌ
10. up	ʌp
11. please	baɪ
12. bye	baɪ
13. bag	baɪ

(continued)

SPEECH SAMPLE *(continued)*

Intended Words	E
14. bubble	bʌ
15. pop	bɑp
16. ball	bɔ
17. Pop Pop*	pɑp pɑp

* = Pop Pop is the family name for grandfather.

QUESTIONS

1. What common error pattern affects E's pronunciation of voiceless oral stops in word initial position?

2. Which word is an apparent exception to this error pattern?

3. Are there environments in which E is able to produce voiceless oral stops? If yes, what is the environment?

4. Suppose you focus on word initial [p] as a treatment target. Answer the following questions about E's better abilities.

   A. What is a possible key word for [p] in word initial position?

   B. What is a possible key environment for [p]?

5. Suppose you wish to test your hypothesis about *Pop Pop* being a key word. You wait for E to pronounce *please, pop,* and *Pop Pop*. Based on the information obtained from those pronunciations, answer the following questions.

   A. If your hypothesis about *Pop Pop* being a key word is right, will [p] in that word be pronounced correctly more often in *Pop Pop* than in the other two words?

   B. Suppose your hypothesis about *Pop Pop* being a key word is incorrect and that, instead, it is only chance that [p] is pronounced correctly in that word rather than in the other two words. If *Pop Pop* is not a key word, will [p] in that word be pronounced correctly more often than in the other words?

Answer Sheet for Exercise 12–2: Better Abilities

1. **Error pattern:**

2. **Exception:**

3.

4. A. **Possible key word:**

   B. **Possible key environment:**

5. A. **Yes/no:**

   B. **Yes/no:**

Exercise 12–3: Better Abilities

This exercise provides another opportunity to perform analyses of key environments and key words. The exercise is based on the speech of Bobby, a child 5 years, 7 months of age who was born and raised in Hawaii (see Appendix C–6 for the complete speech sample). The parental report is unremarkable except for a history of chronic otitis media resulting in placement of bilateral PE tubes during the early preschool years. A hearing screening performed at the time of the speech-language evaluation indicates normal hearing.

Chance? A Word? Or Context?

Suppose that during an initial evaluation a client pronounces [s] incorrectly except in *seat*. Was it just chance that [s] was pronounced correctly in *seat* rather than in some other words? Or is *seat* a key word? Or is word initial position before [i] a key phonetic environment? If chance is responsible for the correct pronunciation of [s], during word probes the client's pronunciation of [s] should be correct no more often in *seat* than in other words. If *seat* is a key word, during word probes the client's pronunciation of [s] should be correct far more often in *seat* than in other words. If *seat* contains a key phonetic environment, during word probes the client's pronunciation of [s] should be correct far more often in those words that contain the same phonetic environment than in other words.

SPEECH SAMPLE

Intended Words	Bobby
11. cake	teɪk
12. car	tɑr
13. carrots	tærɛts
14. cat	tæt
15. cold	toʊd
16. comb	toʊm
17. cornflake	toʊrnfweɪt
18. country	tʌntʃwi
19. cow	taʊ
20. cup	tʌp
21. key	ki
22. king	tɪŋ
23. kiss	tɪs
24. Quick	kwɪk
25. cry	tʃwaɪ

(continued)

SPEECH SAMPLE *(continued)*

Intended Words	Bobby
26. clock	kwɑk
42. get	dɛt
43. girl	gɝl
44. give	dɪv
45. go	doʊ
46. going	doʊ.ɪŋ
47. gum	dʌm
48. gun	dʌn
49. green	gwin
50. grow	gwoʊ
51. glue	gwu

QUESTIONS

1. What is the name of the error pattern that affects the first consonant in *cake, car,* and *carrots*?

2. Is there a first bet for velar consonants? If so, what is it?

3. Is Bobby better able to pronounce velar consonants in the first bet environment?

4. Bobby also demonstrates some ability to pronounce velar consonants in other environments. Is Bobby able to pronounce velar consonants in non-cluster environments in the beginning of any words? If yes, what are the words?

5. *Key* and *girl* might be key words. Alternately, it might simply be chance that Bobby pronounces the velar consonant correctly in these specific words rather than in some other two words. One simple method to help determine if *key* and *girl* are key words is to ask Bobby to pronounce five words beginning with velar consonants, two of which are *key* and *girl*. If *key* and *girl* are key words, what do you expect the results of the word probe to be?

6. What should be the results of the word probe if only chance determines that the velar consonants are correct in *key* and *girl* rather than in other words?

7. Does Bobby demonstrate any ability to pronounce velar consonants in word initial consonant clusters? If so, what are the words?

8. Is word initial consonant clusters a first bet phonetic environment for velar consonants?

9. *For discussion:* Can you develop a phonetic explanation for why word initial consonant clusters is a key environment for Bobby? (**Hint:** Look at both consonants in the word initial consonant clusters).

10. *For discussion:* What do you consider the merits and limitations of the analyses of key environments and key words?

Answer Sheet for Exercise 12–3: Better Abilities

1. **Error pattern:**

2. **First bet:**

3.

4. **Words:**

5. **Key word results:**

6. **Chance results:**

7. **Words:**

8.

9. *For discussion:*

10. *For discussion:*

CHAPTER

13

Related Analyses

with Brian Goldstein

Several analyses are performed in conjunction with the assessments described in the previous three chapters. Possible related analyses include adjusted age, developmental age, dialect, and acquisition strategies.

ADJUSTED AGE

Adjusted age is calculated for clients 24 months or younger who were born prematurely to establish the client's best potential for articulation and phonological development. For example, a client with a chronological age of 22 months and an adjusted age of 20 months is expected to have the articulation and phonological skills of a child 20 months of age, not a child 22 months of age. The formula to determine adjusted age is chronological age in months minus prematurity in months.

DEVELOPMENTAL AGE

Developmental age is calculated for clients with suspected intellectual or cognitive impairments to establish the client's potential for articulation and

---

Hope

Sometimes the results of an assessment indicate a client faces a challenging developmental future. To illustrate, a child brought in for a supposed speech delay may be found to also have severe developmental delays in language reception and cognition. Parents have the right to know their child's likely prognosis for future development. However, when conveying difficult information, also provide some hope. The first step in a parent's journey from a difficult today to a manageable future can be as simple as the name of a good intervention program or the telephone number of a gifted therapist. Hope costs no more than despair, and hope is much easier to live with day to day.

phonological development. For example, a client whose chronological age is 9 years, but whose developmental age is 6 years, is expected to have the articulation and phonological development commensurate to a child 6 years of age. Developmental age is best calculated based on the age corresponding to the client's verbal intelligence. The following formula is used to calculate developmental age. If a verbal intelligence score is unavailable, some clinicians substitute language reception abilities in months for verbal intelligence.

$$\frac{\text{Verbal IQ} \times \text{CA in months}}{100} = \text{Developmental Age}$$

DIALECT

The influence of **dialect** is identified in all appropriate clients in Stages 2 through 4 to distinguish a language difference from a possible articulation and phonological disorder. The dialect patterns of African-American English Vernacular (AAEV) and Spanish-influenced English (SIE) were presented in Chapter 8 and, for convenience, are repeated in Tables 13–1 and 13–2.

ACQUISITION STRATEGIES

Analysis of **acquisition strategies** is undertaken with clients in Stage 2 and less advanced clients in Stage 3 to identify the possible influence of learning style on assessment and treatment. A description of acquisition strategies was provided in Chapter 9 and, for convenience, is summarized in Table 13–3.

TABLE 13–1. Major dialect patterns in African-American English Vernacular (AAEV).

Patterns	Examples
Stopping	
[θ] → [t]	*thought* is *tought*
[ð] → [d]	*this* is *dis*
Place changes between vowels and word finally	
[θ] → [f]	*bath* is *baf*
[ð] → [v]	*bathing* is *baving*
[ŋ] → [n]	*swing* is *swin*
Devoicing at ends of words	
[b] → [p]	*slab* is *slap*
[d] → [t]	*bed* is *bet*
[g] → [k]	*bug* is *buk*
Raising of [ɛ] before nasals	
[ɛ] → [ɪ]	*pen* is *pin*
Deletion	
V+ [r] → V + ∅	*more* is *mo*
CC# → C∅#	*nest* is *nes*
Vowel nasalization and nasal deletion	
V + N → nasalized vowel	*tame* is *tã*

Compiled from "Performance of Working Class African American Children on Three Tests of Articulation," Cole & Taylor, 1990, *Language, Speech, and Hearing Services in Schools, 21*, 171–176.

TABLE 13–2. Characteristics of Spanish-influenced English (SIE).

Patterns	Examples
Affrication	
/ʃ/ → [tʃ]	/fɪʃ/ → [fɪtʃ]
/j/ → [dʒ]	/jɛlo/ → [dʒɛlo]
Consonant Devoicing	
/z/ → [s]	/hɪz/ → [hɪs]
/dʒ/ → [tʃ]	/dʒɛl/ → [tʃɛl]
Nasal Velarization	
/n/ → [ŋ]	/fæn/ → [fæŋ]
Stopping	
/v/ → [b]	/ves/ → [bes]
/θ/ → [t]	/θət/ → [tat]
/ð/ → [d]	/ðo/ → [do]

Compiled from "Dialectal variations," by A. Iglesias & N. Anderson, 1993. In J. Bernthal & N. Bankson (Eds.), *Articulation and phonological disorders*, (3rd ed., pp. 147–161). New York: Prentice-Hall.

TABLE 13–3. Major articulation and phonological acquisition strategies.

Strategies	Hallmark
Regressions	The client temporarily loses a speech ability. A temporary regression may last from days to months.
Favorite sounds	The client uses a sound (sometimes an unusual one, such as syllabic [s]) in place of many other sounds.
Selectivity	The client "picks and chooses" words that contain sounds and sound sequences that he or she already produces.
Word recipes	The client's words are organized into a few sound patterns.
Homonyms	The client either avoids or seeks words that are pronounced as homonyms
Word-based learning	The client's pronunciation of a sound varies depending on the word in which it occurs.
Gestalt learning	The client knows "the tune before the words."

Exercise 13–1: Related Analyses

Adjusted and developmental age are simple, but important calculations performed for certain groups of clients. This exercise provides opportunities to practice these calculations, and, more importantly, to explore the rationale that underlies their use.

QUESTIONS

1. Suppose a client is born 3 months prematurely. What is the client's adjusted age when the toddler is 1 year, 6 months of age?

2. What is the client's adjusted age at 2 years, 3 months of age?

3. Why do you suppose adjusted age is calculated for children born prematurely?

4. Why do you suppose adjusted age is not calculated for children over 2 years, 0 months of age?

5. Suppose a client is born with Down syndrome, and that an intelligence test administered at 3 years, 11 months of age estimates his or her intelligence to be 57. What is the client's developmental age?

6. Suppose that at 3 years, 11 months of age the above client's articulation and phonological development approximates that of a child near 2 years, 2 months of age. Does the client have an articulation and phonological disorder? Why or why not?

7. Sometimes an intelligence quotient cannot be obtained, especially with younger children. In such situations, clinicians typically compare the client's articulation and phonological development to his or her language reception abilities. Suppose a client who is 4 years, 4 months of age has language reception abilities that approximate those of a child near 2 years, 0 months to 2 years, 4 months of age. The client's articulation and phonological abilities also approximate a child near 2 years, 0 months to 2 years, 4 months of age. Does this client have an articulation and phonological disorder?

8. *For discussion:* What do you consider the merits and limitations of the concept of developmental age?

Answer Sheet for Exercise 13–1: Related Analyses

1. **Adjusted age:**

2. **Adjusted age:**

3. **Rationale:**

4.

5.   _____X_____ =

6.

7.

8. *For discussion:*

Exercise 13–2: Related Analyses

A multitude of dialects exist in the United States. Each clinician has the responsibility to know the dialect patterns of the communities in which a given client resides. This exercise focuses on dialect patterns in the speech of a client 4 years, 0 months of age who speaks a variety of African American English Vernacular (AAEV) (Goldstein, 1995). Additionally, the present exercise affords an opportunity to consider issues that arise in sentence elicitation tasks such as those used in the sentence subtest of the *Goldman-Fristoe Test of Articulation* (Goldman & Fristoe, 1969).

SPEECH SAMPLE

Client's Sentences

1. Jerry is playing with his drum, ball, and wagon.
   dɛri ɪs plejin wɪf hɪs dʌm al en wædĩ
2. He is making too much noise.
   ʔi ɪ metin tũ muʃ nɔɪ
3. His mother makes him stop.
   hɪz mʌdɚ met hĩ tap
4. It is time to take a bath.
   ʔɪ ʔɪ tãɪ du tet e væf
5. Oh, no! He loses the soap.
   o no hi lu də sot

QUESTIONS

1. Complete the following table, identifying the client's AAEV patterns and possible articulation and phonological errors. For convenience, the client's sentences are included on the answer sheet. Indicate possible articulation and phonological errors using the X/Y notation described in Chapter 4. *The first sentence is an example and is answered for you.*

2. *For discussion:* The speech sample for this exercise was elicited by having the client describe a series of pictures. What do you consider the values and limitations of analyzing a client's production of sentences using a picture description task?

Answer Sheet for Exercise 13–2: Related Analyses

1. **Sentences:**

   (1) Jerry is playing with his drum, ball, and wagon.
       dɛri ɪs plejin wɪf hɪs dʌm al en wædĩ
       AAEV Pattern(s): Place Change (n/ŋ in *playing*)
                             Place Change (f/θ in *with*)
                             Vowel Nasalization & Deletion (in *wagon*)
       Errors: d/dʒ (*Jerry*)
                 d/dr (*drum*)
                 ɸ/b (*ball*)
                 d/g (in *wagon*)

   (2) He is making too much noise.
       ʔi ɪ metin tũ mu nɔɪ
       AAEV Pattern(s):
       Errors:

   (3) His mother makes him stop.
       hɪz mʌdɚ met hĩ tap
       AAEV Pattern(s):
       Errors:

   (4) It is time to take a bath.
       ʔɪ ʔɪ tãɪ du tet e væf
       AAEV Pattern(s):
       Errors:

   (5) Oh, no! He loses the soap.
       o no hi lu də sot
       AAEV Pattern(s):
       Errors:

2. *For discussion:*

Exercise 13–3: Related Analyses

Clinicians who work with clients who speak SIE must be able to distinguish dialect patterns from possible developmental errors. This exercise considers dialect patterns and possible developmental errors in the speech of child 4 years of age who is a speaker of SIE (Goldstein, 1995).

The Role of the Monolingual Clinician

Monolingual clinicians sometimes find themselves in the position of deciding whether or not it is appropriate to treat communication disorders in children who are learning English as a second language. To provide such care, the clinician's knowledge base needs to include, but not be limited to, information on placement options, state and federal laws, first and second language acquisition, and culturally sensitive assessment and treatment techniques. A primary task of the clinician during the evaluation is to differentiate second language acquisition patterns from errors indicating possible articulation and phonological disorders—a difficult task under any conditions, but one made even more challenging if (as often is the case) little information exists on the child's first language and its dialects. Monolingual clinicians, while having a role in the client's assessment, need not serve as a direct service provider. Rather, the clinician's role may be that of a consultant or advocate who works in conjunction with a bilingual clinician or interpreter.

SPEECH SAMPLE

Intended Words	Child
1. pencils	[kɛnsɪls]
2. matches	[nates]
3. drum	[drʌt]
4. duck	[dʌt]
5. shovel	[tʃʌbəl]
6. rabbit	[rabit]
7. carrot	[kæwɪt]
8. pajama	[pitʃama]
9. orange	[orintʃ]
10. stove	[sob]
11. feather	[felo]
12. blue	[bu]

PROBLEM

Complete the table on the answer sheet, identifying differences between English and the client's speech and indicating whether the differences are the result of SIE or possible developmental errors. (*Hint:* More than one SIE pattern and developmental error can affect the same word, and words can contain both multiple SIE patterns and developmental errors.) *The first word is an example and is answered for you.*

Answer Sheet for Exercise 13–3: Related Analyses

Intended Words	Child	SIE	Errors
1. pencils	[kɛnsɪls]	Consonant Devoicing	p → k
2. matches	[nates]		
3. drum	[drʌt]		
4. duck	[dʌt]		
5. shovel	[tʃʌbəl]		
6. rabbit	[rabit]		

(continued)

Intended Words	Child	SIE	Errors
(continued)			
7. carrot	[kæwɪt]		
8. pajama	[pitʃama]		
9. orange	[orintʃ]		
10. stove	[sob]		
11. feather	[felo]		
12. blue	[bu]		

Exercise 13–4: Related Analyses

The full range of acquisition strategies found in the speech of typically developing children also occur in the speech of persons with articulation and phonological disorders. The information for this exercise comes from E, the child whose speech was described in several exercises in previous chapters. As described previously, E was born prematurely, and received a tracheostomy when she was approximately 3 months of age subsequent to bronchopul- monary dysplasia (BPD), a lung problem sometimes resulting from medical efforts to save children whose immature lungs are too weak to provide the breaths of life (Bleile, Stark, & Silverman McGowan, 1993). E's tracheostomy tube was removed when she was 2 years, 4 months of age. The following words are E's entire expressive vocabulary at 2 years, 8 months of age.

SPEECH SAMPLE

Intended Words	E
1. daddy	dædə
2. hi	haɪ
3. down	da
4. mom	mɑm
5. hop	bɑp
6. water	wɑwa
7. book	bʊk
8. bow	boʊ
9. baby	bʌbʌ
10. up	ʌp
11. please	baɪ
12. bye	baɪ
13. bag	baɪ
14. bubble	bʌ
15. pop	bɑp
16. ball	bɔ
17. Pop Pop*	pɑp pɑp

* = Pop Pop is the family name for grandfather.

QUESTIONS

1. A total of 16 of 17 words that E attempted begin with consonants. Identify how many of these consonants are produced at each place of production. For example, if four words begin with postalveolar consonants then postalveolar = 4. (*Hint:* For this exercise cover E's pronunciation and only consider the words E attempts.)

2. Convert your answer from the first question into a percentage value for bilabial consonants.

3. Compare your answer to the percentage values for bilabial consonants displayed in Table 10–3, which shows the approximate relative frequency of English consonants. According to that table, what percentage of English consonants are bilabial?

4. Identify and describe E's acquisition strategy based on your answers to the first three questions.

5. *For discussion:* Why might E have developed such a strategy?

Answer Sheet for Exercise 13–4: Related Analyses

1. **Bilabial Alveolar Glottal**

2. **Bilabial =**

3. **Expected relative frequency =   %**

4. **Strategy:**

5. *For discussion:*

Exercise 13–5: Related Analyses

This exercise focuses on another type of acquisition strategy in the speech of a client with an articulation and phonological disorder. The client is named Mike, a Korean child who was adopted by an American couple when he was 2 years, 2 months of age.

Mike is approximately 4 years, 8 months of age (Pollack, 1983). The words constitute Mike's entire expressive vocabulary. Cognitive and receptive language testing indicate he is functioning within age-normal limits.

Mike

Karen Pollock, the author of the original study of Mike's speech, reestablished contact with Mike's family when he was 17 years of age. Mike's mother reported that Mike spoke well, but that when he became tired some of the old speech errors would return. She also recalled that Mike had received speech therapy through elementary school, but that he had made the most progress around 4th and 5th grade when she felt peer pressure appeared to help motivate him to improve.

SPEECH SAMPLE

Intended Words	Mike
1. balls	da
2. dish	dɪ
3. hat	næ
4. fast	dæ
5. got	da
6. mask	næ
7. stand	dæ
8. sun	da~ dan
9. right	na
10. tent	dɛ

QUESTIONS

1. Spend a minute considering Mike's speech. (*Hint:* Sometimes you can obtain a better grasp of a client's speech by saying words as the client says them.) *This item does not require a written answer.*

2. Did you notice that Mike's phonetic inventory is very restricted? Which acquisition strategy describes groups of words that a child produces in a few simple ways? (*Hint:* For this exercise focus on Mike's pronunciations rather than the words he attempts.)

3. Mike's speech appears to contain two word recipes. What are the numbers of the words that belong to the recipe that includes the first word? (*Hint:* The third word belongs to the other word recipe.)

4. What are the numbers of the words that belong to the recipe that includes the third word?

5. The phonetic inventories of both word recipes are similar. Describe the similarities between the word recipes in terms of stress, sequence of syllables, and consonant distinctive features. (*Hint:* Ignore the alternate pronunciation of *sun* as [dan], which appears to be an exception.)

6. The two word recipes differ in several ways. Describe the differences in terms of consonants and consonant distinctive features.

Answer Sheet for Exercise 13–5: Related Analyses

1. **(no answer)**

2. **Strategy:**

3. **Word numbers:**

4. **Word numbers:**

5. **Stress:**
   Sequence of syllables:
   Consonant distinctive features:

6. **Consonants:**
   Consonant distinctive features:

SECTION
IV

Treatment Principles

OVERVIEW

Treatment is the heart of the clinical enterprise. The exercises in this section examine the treatment principles that underlie selection of long- and short-term goals, treatment targets, administrative decisions, and treatment progress assessment. A special feature of this section is a series of exercises that describe treatment decisions for three clients from goal selection through treatment progress assessment. The clients were chosen because they represent a range of articulation and phonological development rather than because they are "typical." (I am not sure what constitutes a typical articulation and phonological disorder.)

Why Treatment?

In this world with all its problems, aren't there better things for people and societies to spend time and money on than helping people speak better? My own answer to this question is that the implications of a speech problem, rather than the speech problems themselves, justify the need for treatment. Speech is not a luxury—rather, speech is how we think, negotiate, tell stories, joke, make friends, argue, and make up. Speech is a tie that binds people together, and a person with a speech problem is someone for whom this tie is loosened.

CHAPTER
14

Goals

Long-term goals are the articulation and phonological behaviors that a client is expected to exhibit either at the end of treatment or after a designated time period, such as a semester or school year. Long-term goals may differ depending on whether the client has intellectual or cognitive impairments or was born prematurely.

For clients without cognitive or intellectual impairments, the most common long-term goal is for articulation and phonological development to be appropriate to the client's chronological age. For clients with cognitive or intellectual impairments, the most common long-term goal is for articulation and phonological development to be appropriate to the client's language reception abilities. For clients under 2 years old who were born prematurely, the most common long-term goal is for articulation and phonological development to be appropriate to the client's adjusted age, which is the client's chronological age minus the months born prematurely. Lastly, a possible long-term goal for all clients is to eliminate articulation and phonological errors that influence a person's happiness or social and educational development. Such a long-term goal is appropriate, for example, for a client who was teased because of a [w] for [r] substitution or who experienced embarrassment when speaking to groups because of a frontal lisp.

Short-term goals are the steps, each typically lasting from a few weeks to several months, through which long-term goals are achieved. The major short-term goals for clients at the four stages in articulation and phonological development are listed in Table 14–1.

REDUCE HOMONYMS

This short-term goal seeks to reduce the percentage of homonyms (words that sound alike, but have dif-

TABLE 14–1. Short-term goals for clients at three stages of articulation and phonological development.

Stages	Short-Term Goal
Stage 2 and 3	• Reduction in homonyms • Reduction of variability • Maximization of established speech ability • Elimination of errors affecting sound classes
Stage 4	• Facilitation of late-acquired consonants, consonant clusters, and unstressed syllables in more difficult multisyllabic words

ferent meanings) in a client's speech. There are two general approaches to reducing homonyms: **eliminate errors causing homonyms** and **flooding**. The first approach, as its name implies, seeks to eliminate error patterns or sound class errors causing homonyms (Ingram, 1989). A client, for example, who pronounced *cookie*, *Tom*, *kite*, and *toe* as [di] might have reduction of Fronting as a short-term goal, so that *cookie* and *kite* would then be pronounced with an initial [k] and *Tom* and *toe* would be pronounced with an initial [t].

The second approach, **flooding**, seeks to reduce the number of homonyms by causing the client to reorganize his or her articulation and phonological systems (Bleile & Miller, 1994). Somewhat ironically, flooding works by facilitating the acquisition of words that result in an increased number of homonyms in a client's speech. The increase in the number of homonyms results in communicative breakdown and frustration, inducing speech changes as the client is forced to attempt new pronunciations to communicate. Flooding is an experimental procedure. Within a flooding approach, a client whose expressive vocabulary was dominated by words pronounced as [di], for example, would be taught words that the assessment indicated would also be pronounced [di]. The clinician would then engage the client in the type of request for clarification activities described in Chapter 21. To illustrate, the client might say [di] as a request for a cookie, and the clinician might give him or her a spoon, key, or plate, or other object that the client also pronounces as [di].

REDUCE VARIABILITY

This short-term goal seeks to reduce a client's alternate pronunciations of words and sounds. Reduction in variability is appropriate for clients in Stage 2 and some less advanced clients in Stage 3 who appear extremely variable in their pronunciation of a sound or sounds.

There are two types of variability: **intraword variability** and **interword variability**. Intraword variability is variation in the pronunciation of a sound or sounds in the same word. A client whose speech showed intraword variability, for example, might say the initial sound in *bee* as [b], [p], or [mb]. Interword variability is variation in the pronunciation of a sound or sounds in different words. A client whose speech showed interword variability, for example, might say [b] as [b] in *bee*, as [d] in *bay*, and as [p] in *boo*.

Both intra- and inter-word variability interferes with communication. More positively, however,

variability suggests that better pronunciation of a sound is within the client's phonetic abilities, even though the client may not yet be able to produce it correctly on all occasions. When the short-term goal is to reduce variability, the general clinical strategy is to use facilitative techniques that encourage the client to produce the most developmentally advanced variant of the sound.

MAXIMIZE ESTABLISHED SPEECH ABILITIES

This short-term goal seeks to maximize a client's existing articulation and phonological abilities (Bleile & Miller, 1994). Maximizing established speech abilities is appropriate for clients in Stage 2 for whom the major treatment goal is vocabulary building and less advanced clients in Stage 3 who are temporarily "stalled" in articulation and phonological development. This short-term goal involves increasing the use of the client's existing abilities to pronounce sounds, syllables, and word shapes. Use of established speech abilities reduces the speech complexity of learning new words, particularly if the client's speech is organized around word recipes or selectivity (see Chapter 9). The constructed words should be pragmatically useful and contain well-established sounds, syllables, and word shapes. If the client's established phonetic inventory, for example, contains the CV syllables, [k], and [i], the clinician would discuss with the client's parents whether the word *key* has functional value for the client. If so, *key* would receive special emphasis during treatment and the client's family would be encouraged to facilitate use of the word at home.

ELIMINATE ERRORS AFFECTING SOUND CLASSES

This short-term goal seeks to eliminate errors that affect entire classes of sounds. All clients in Stages 2 and 3 whose speech contains articulation and phonological errors affecting sound classes are appropriate candidates for elimination of the errors. Two closely related approaches are used to eliminate errors affecting sound classes: distinctive feature approaches and error pattern approaches.

Distinctive Feature Approaches

In a **distinctive feature approach**, sounds are remediated based on their membership in a sound class.

The sound classes most often used for this purpose are the various place, manner, and voicing categories found in a consonant chart. Some clinicians remediate all sounds in a sound class (Blodgett & Miller, 1989). For example, a clinician might treat all velar consonants in the speech of a client who pronounced velar consonants as alveolar consonants. Other clinicians recommend treating fewer sounds within a sound class (Elbert, Powell, & Swartzlander, 1991; Williams, 1991). My own approach is to remediate from two sounds up to 50% of the sounds in a sound class in the hope that the treatment results will generalize to other sounds sharing the distinctive feature. For example, treatment for a client who pronounced [k] and [g] as alveolar consonants in the beginning of syllables might focus on facilitating acquisition of [k] in the hope that the client will generalize the ability to produce stop consonants in the velar region to other velar consonants. The motivation for remediating only a few sounds in a sound class is that it saves time for the clients who generalize and costs no additional time for those who do not.

Error Pattern Approaches

An **error pattern approach** seeks to eliminate sounds based on their membership in error patterns. As with the distinctive feature approach, some clinicians provide treatment to all sounds affected by an error pattern; whereas others, the author included, remediate from two sounds up to 50% of the sounds affected by an error pattern in the hope that the treatment results will generalize to other sounds affected by the error pattern. A client, for example, might have a Fronting error pattern in the beginning of syllables, and treatment might focus on remediating [k] in that syllable position in the hope that the results will generalize to [g].

An important issue to consider is which error patterns should be selected for remediation. Table 14–2 offers a simple means to categorize error patterns according to their prevalence. I typically select error patterns for remediation that are either frequent (50%–75% of all possible occurrences) or present (25%–49% of all occurrences), and tend to avoid error patterns that are highly frequent (75%–100% of all possible occurrences), because their remediation often is too time-consuming for younger clients. I also tend to avoid remediating error patterns that are disappearing (1%–24%), because in most situations the client appears to be overcoming them without treatment.

INDIVIDUAL CONSONANTS, CONSONANT CLUSTERS, MULTISYLLABIC WORDS

The major short-term goal for clients in Stage 4 is to facilitate the elimination of errors affecting late-acquired consonants, consonant clusters, and unstressed syllables in more difficult multisyllabic words. A client, for example, might be limited to word-initial syllables beginning with a consonant (C) followed by a vowel (V). A possible goal for such a client would be to facilitate the acquisition of syllables that begin with consonant clusters (Bernhardt, in press; Bernhardt & Gilbert, 1992). Table 14–3 offers a simple means to categorize sounds according to the frequency with which they are pronounced correctly. Most often, emerging (10%–49% correct) sounds and syllables are selected as short-term goals. However, rare (1%–9% correct) sounds and syllables are sometimes selected as short-term goals for clients who are capable of overcoming frustration, and acquired (50%–74% correct) sounds and syllables are sometimes selected with clients who

TABLE 14–2. Percentage and whole number criteria for disappearance of error patterns.

Categories	Percentages	Whole Numbers* (5 Chances)	Whole Numbers (10 Chances)
Highly frequent	75% to 100%	4/5–5/5	8/10–10/10
Frequent	50% to 74%	3/5	5/10–7/10
Present	25% to 49%	2/5	3/10–4/10
Disappearing	1% to 24%	1/5	1/10–2/10
Disappeared	0%	0/5	0/10

* = Whole numbers are the number of different words. For example, 3/5 means the error pattern occurred in 3 of 5 words.

Which Table?

Which table to use (Table 14–2 or 14–3) depends largely on a client's stage in articulation and phonological development. Table 14–2 is generally used with clients in Stage 2 and 3, and Table 14–3 is generally used with clients in Stage 4. It is possible, however, to use both tables with clients in Stage 2 and 3. To illustrate, a clinician might use Table 14–2 to determine how often an error pattern occurs and use Table 14–3 to determine how often sounds affected by error patterns are pronounced correctly.

TABLE 14–3. Percentage and whole number criteria for acquisition of consonants and consonant clusters.

Categories	Percentages	Whole Numbers (5 Chances)	Whole Numbers (10 Chances)
Mastered	75% to 100%	4/5-5/5	8/10–10/10
Acquired	50% to 74%	3/5	5/10–7/10
Emerging	25% to 49%	2/5	3/10–4/10
Rare	1% to 24%	1/5	1/10–2/10
Absent	0%	0/5	0/10

* = Whole numbers are the number of different words. For example, 4/5 means the sound was produced correctly in 4 of 5 words.

do not appear to be improving without treatment. Absent (0% correct) sounds and syllables are seldom selected as short-term goals, because they often prove extremely challenging for clients; mastered (75%–100% correct) sounds and syllables are seldom selected because they appear well on the way to already being acquired.

Exercise 14–1: Goals

The selection of long-term goals is affected by such factors as the client's age, cognitive development, and social concerns. This exercise provides practice in writing long-term goals for a variety of clients.

Attached to Every Speech Problem . . .

How do you decide between alternative goals and treatment targets? For example, when do you select reduction of homonyms as a short-term goal and when elimination of errors affecting sound classes? In some situations, the analysis of a speech sample yields a clear preference between possible choices. However, attached to every speech problem is a real human being, and treatment decisions need to include such human factors as what sounds cause the client to be teased and what sounds concern the client and his or her family.

QUESTIONS

1. Write a long-term goal for a 4-year-old girl who is without cognitive or intellectual impairments. *This is an example and is answered for you.*

2. Write a long-term goal for a client 6 years, 7 months of age who is mentally retarded.

3. Write a long-term goal for a client 18 months of age who was born 3 months prematurely. The client has no intellectual or cognitive impairments.

4. Write a long-term goal for a client 25 months of age who was born 2 months prematurely. The client is without intellectual or cognitive impairments.

5. Write a long-term goal for a client 13 years of age who has no intellectual or cognitive impairments.

6. Write a long-term goal for a client 13 months of age who was born 2 months prematurely and whose cognitive development approximates that of a child aged 6 months of age.

7. Write a long-term goal for a client 20 months of age who was born 3 months prematurely and whose cognitive development approximates that of a child aged 17 months of age.

8. Write a long-term goal for a client 7 years of age who has no intellectual and cognitive impairments and has been accepted into treatment because teasing about his [w] for [r] pattern.

Answer Sheet for Exercise 14–1: Goals

1. **Long-term goal:** The long-term goal is for the client's articulation and phonological development to be appropriate to her chronological age.

2. **Long-term goal:**

3. **Long-term goal:**

4. **Long-term goal:**

5. **Long-term goal:**

6. **Long-term goal:**

7. **Long-term goal:**

8. **Long-term goal:**

Exercise 14–2: Goals

Selecting a short-term goal or goals is an important clinical decision that must be made for every client. This exercise asks you to match a statement that best corresponds to one of the many possible short-term goals for clients in Stages 2 and 3.

Keep Your Eyes on the Prize

Most error patterns produce poor short term goals. Some occur so rarely that a client will likely eliminate the patterns without assistance, others occur so regularly that the clinician has little immediate chance to affect them. Instead of trying to analyze all the error patterns in a client's speech, keep your eyes on the prize, giving your attention to those aspects of the speech sample through which you may contribute to a person's articulation and phonological development.

QUESTIONS

1. Which short-term goal is reduction in variability in how a sound is produced in a number of different words? *This is an example and is answered for you.*

2. Maximization of the client's expressive vocabulary through the use of sounds and syllables already in the client's phonetic inventory is which short-term goal?

3. Which short-term goal should lead to reduction in homonyms through treatment of the error patterns causing the child to pronounce words similarly?

4. The short-term goal for reduction in the error patterns affecting a client's speech is what?

5. Reduction in variability of a sound in a word is which short-term goal?

6. Reduction in homonyms through a language-based approach designed to facilitate a client's reorganization of his or her articulation and phonological system could be which short-term goal?

7. Which short-term goal involves facilitation of the client's acquisition of distinctive features?

Answer Sheet for Exercise 14–2: Goals

1. **Short-term goal:** reduction in interword variability

2. **Short-term goal:**

3. **Short-term goal:**

4. **Short-term goal:**

5. **Short-term goal:**

6. **Short-term goal:**

7. **Short-term goal:**

Exercise 14–3: Short-term Goals

Several short-term goals, especially those for clients in Stage 2 and 3, involve analytical decisions somewhat different than those encountered in previous sections. This exercise focuses on reduction of homonyms. The speech sample on which this exercise is based is from Tommy, a 5-year-old boy with Down syndrome (Bodine, 1974).

SPEECH SAMPLE

Intended Words	Tommy
1. piece	bi
2. please	bi
3. B	bi
4. big	bi
5. talk	da
6. Kathy	da
7. coffee	da
8. Jack	da
9. jacket	da
10. that	da
11. chocolate	da

QUESTIONS

1. Suppose you select reduction of homonyms as your short-term goal, and you choose to accomplish this goal through eliminating errors causing homonyms. Answer the following questions about the error patterns that affect the first four words. (**Hint:** This and the following questions ask you to analyze error patterns; the questions could also be answered through analysis of distinctive features.)

   A. What error patterns affect word initial consonants? *This is an example and is answered for you.*
   B. What error pattern affects word final consonants?
   C. What error pattern affects vowels? (**Hint:** The error pattern that affects vowels is uncommon and does not have a name.)

2. Perform the same analysis for words 5 through 11.

   A. What error patterns affect word initial consonants?
   B. What error patterns affect word final consonants?
   C. What error pattern affects vowels? (*Hint:* The simplest way to describe this error pattern is to list the vowels that Tommy pronounces as [a].)

3. *For discussion:* Which error pattern or error patterns would you select as short-term goals to reduce the number of homonyms in Tommy's speech?

4. Flooding is an alternative approach to eliminating homonyms in a client's speech. Within a flooding approach, the clinician selects words to teach that the client is likely to pronounce as homonyms. Based on your analysis of Tommy's homonyms, list two words that Tommy would likely pronounce as [bi] and two words that he would likely pronounce as [da].

5. *For discussion:* What are the similarities and differences between the two short-term goals to reduce homonyms?

Answer Sheet for Exercise 14–3: Goals

1. A. **Error pattern:** Prevocalic Voicing (1–4)

   Cluster Reduction (2)

   B. **Error pattern:**
   C. **Error pattern:**

2. A. **Error patterns:**
   B. **Error patterns:**
   C. **Error pattern:**

3. *For discussion:*

4. [bi]:

   [da]:

5. *For discussion:*

Exercise 14–4: Goals

This exercise addresses decisions involving long- and short-term goals for Gavin, a client in Stage 2 who is 4 years, 8 months of age. Results of a battery of language and psychological tests indicate that Gavin's cognitive development approximates that of a child near 3 years of age.

Answers Can (and Should) Vary

Rather than presenting "correct" treatment principles, the purpose in discussing Gavin, Kelly, and Billy is to describe a logical basis for making clinical decisions. Your answers to the exercise questions in this and the following chapters are likely to differ from those in the appendix. It is far more important to develop a strong clinical rationale for clinical decisions than to agree with the answers in this or any other book.

SPEECH SAMPLE

See Appendix C–3.

QUESTIONS

1. Provide a long-term goal for Gavin's articulation and phonological treatment.

2. What are the major options for short-term goals for clients in Gavin's stage in articulation and phonological development?

3. Does homonym reduction seem a plausible short-term goal for Gavin? Why or why not? (**Hint:** Clinical care seldom affords the time for in-depth analyses of each possible short-term goal. This and the following questions ask you to present your initial hypothesis rather than to perform careful analyses for each potential short-term goal.) *This is an example and is answered for you.*

4. Does reduction in variability seem a plausible short-term goal for Gavin? Why or why not? (**Hint:** Focus your analysis on words in which a variant is a "correct" sound.)

5. Does maximization of established speech abilities seem a plausible short-term goal for Gavin? Why or why not?

6. Does elimination of errors affecting sound classes seem a plausible short-term goal for Gavin? Why or why not? (**Hint:** Focus on those error patterns that seem the best candidates to be short-term goals, identifying only those error patterns that affect 3 or more words, setting aside error patterns that contain sounds never pronounced correctly even variably, and counting sounds produced variably as being produced incorrectly.)

7. *For discussion:* Which of the short-term goal or goals do you select for Gavin?

Answer Sheet for Exercise 14–4: Goals

1. **Long-term goal:**

2. **Options for short-term goals:**

3. **Reduce homonyms:** Yes. Gavin's speech contains a number of homonyms. Two particularly common homonyms are [bʌ] and [dʌ]. The error pattern giving rise to the homonyms is described in answer to a question that follows.

4. **Reduce variability:**

5. **Maximize established speech abilities:**

6. **Elimination of errors affecting sound classes:**

7. *For discussion:*

Exercise 14–5: Goals

This exercise addresses decisions regarding long- and short-term goals for Kelly, a client in Stage 3 who was born 2 months prematurely. Kelly is 5 years, 10 months of age and is doing well in a regular classroom.

Clinical Tools

Word probes are short (five to ten words) lists of words that are used to assess development and as treatment pre- and posttests. There are two types of word probes: **error probes** and **sound probes**. Error probes help determine the extent to which error patterns exist, and sound probes help determine the extent to which individual sounds and consonant clusters are produced correctly. Both types of word probes are valuable clinical tools because they are flexible, easy to use, and can be administered quickly—three important aspects in any busy clinical setting.

SPEECH SAMPLE

See Appendix C–7.

QUESTIONS

1. Describe a possible long-term goal for Kelly's articulation and phonological treatment.

2. The major options for short-term goals are the same for Kelly as they are for Gavin, including reduce homonyms, reduce variability, maximize established speech abilities, and eliminate errors affecting sound classes. Does reducing homonyms seem a plausible short-term goal for Kelly? Why or why not? *This is an example and is answered for you.*

3. Does reduction in variability seem a plausible short-term goal for Kelly? Why or why not?

4. Does maximization of established speech abilities seem a plausible short-term goal for Kelly? Why or why not?

5. Does elimination of errors affecting sound classes seem a plausible short-term goal for Kelly? Why or why not?

6. Typically, an error probe of five to ten words provides the quickest means to determine frequency of occurrence of error patterns. The results of a hypothetical error probe are shown on the answer sheet. Categorize each of the error patterns according to the system shown in Table 14–2.

7. *For discussion:* Which of the four error patterns would you select as short-term goals?

Answer Sheet for Exercise 14–5: Goals

1. **Long-term goal:**

2. **Reduce homonyms:** No. Kelly's speech sample contains only a few homonyms. For example, *star* and *saw* are homonyms.

3. **Reduce variability:**

4. **Maximize established speech abilities:**

5. **Elimination of errors affecting sound classes:**

6. **Stopping (7/10) =**

   Gliding (6/10) =
   Cluster Reduction (8/10) =
   Affrication (2/5) =

7. *For discussion:*

Exercise 14–6: Goals

This exercise addresses decisions involving long- and short-term goals for Billy, a client in Stage 4 who is 6 years, 8 months of age. Billy is a gifted child who does well at school, but whose speech sometimes causes him to be teased.

SPEECH SAMPLE

See Appendix C–8.

QUESTIONS

1. The brief background on Billy suggests at least two possible long-term goals. What are they?

2. What are the major options for short-term goals for clients in Billy's stage in articulation and phonological development?

3. Does elimination of errors affecting late-acquired consonants seem a plausible short-term goal for Billy? Why or why not? (*Hint:* As with the error pattern analysis, identify errors affecting three or more words, setting aside errors that always occurred, and counting sounds produced variably as being produced incorrectly. For this and the following two questions, determine percentage of occurrence for sounds affected by errors.)

4. Does elimination of errors affecting consonant clusters seem a plausible short-term goal for Billy? Why or why not?

5. Does elimination of errors affecting unstressed syllables in more difficult multisyllabic words seem a plausible short-term goal for Billy? Why or why not?

6. Word probes for [r] in word initial clusters and nonclusters were obtained because the clinician considered these to be likely short-term goals. Results of the word probes indicated [r] was pronounced correctly 28% of the time outside of consonant clusters and 20% of the time in consonant clusters (see Exercise 11–6 for results of the noncluster word probe). To which category does [r] belong according to the system shown in Table 14–3?

7. *For discussion:* Which errors would you select as short-term goals for Billy?

Answer Sheet for Exercise 14–6: Goals

1. **First possible long-term goal:**
   Second possible long-term goal:

2. **Short-term goal:**

3. **Late-acquired consonants:**

4. **Consonant clusters:**

5. **Unstressed syllables:**

6. **Word initial (nonclusters):**
   Word initial (in clusters):

7. *For discussion:*

CHAPTER
15

Treatment Targets

While long- and short-term goals give direction to clinical endeavors, **treatment targets** are the actual sounds and syllables through which change in a client's articulation and phonological systems is facilitated. For example, a long-term goal might be, "Articulation and phonological development will be appropriate for the client's age," and the short-term goal might be, "Elimination of Fronting in the beginning of syllables." The treatment target is the sound (or sounds) through which the restriction on velar consonants (Fronting) in syllable-initial position is eliminated. To illustrate, the clinician might choose [k] as the treatment target, hoping that the results of treating [k] will generalize to other velar consonants. The major issues that arise in considering treatment targets include selecting treatment targets, deciding between most and least knowledge methods, determining how many treatment targets should be treated, changing treatment targets, and choosing linguistic levels and phonetic environments.

SELECTING TREATMENT TARGETS

Most often, the clinician selects treatment targets that the client demonstrates some capacity to produce. Four possible methods to determine if a client is able to produce a treatment target are described in this section and summarized in Table 15–1.

TABLE 15–1. Four methods to select treatment targets.

Criteria	Definitions
Stimulability	The client is stimulable for the treatment target.
Emerging sound	The client can produce the treatment target in either several phonetic environments or one key phonetic environment.
Key word	The client can produce the treatment target in one or a few selected words.
Phonetic placement	The client can produce the treatment target and shaping through phonetic placement or through shaping an existing sound.

Stimulability

Stimulability is the client's ability to imitate a treatment target. Stimulability indicates that a client is physically able to produce the sound. Treatment seeks to generalize use of the sound from imitation to spontaneous speech.

Emerging Sound

An **emerging sound** is one that is produced correctly on 10% to 49% of all occasions in one or more phonetic environments (the phonetic environment is called a **key environment** if the client is only able to produce the treatment target in a single phonetic environment). An example of an emerging sound is [k] in the speech of a client who correctly produced [k] in 3 of 10 words (30%). If the client is able to produce a treatment target in several phonetic environments, treatment seeks to increase the frequency with which the sound is produced. If the client is only able to produce the sound in one key environment, treatment seeks to generalize success from that phonetic environment to other phonetic environments.

Three Stacks

Think of sounds and syllables as belonging in stacks when selecting treatment targets to facilitate new articulation and phonological abilities. The first stack contains sounds and syllables the client always produces correctly; set aside this stack, as the client already produces these sounds and syllables correctly. The second stack contains sounds and syllables the client never produces correctly. The sounds and syllables in this stack are possible but not likely treatment targets, because the client shows no capacity to produce them, and, therefore, is likely to be frustrated if they are selected.

The third stack contains sounds and syllables the client sometimes produces correctly. This is the stack from which you are most likely to select treatment targets, because it contains the sounds and syllables the client shows some capacity to produce, but which he or she cannot produce accurately on all occasions. The sounds and syllables in this stack are those that are emerging, for which the client is stimulable, occur in key words, or can be produced in response to phonetic placement and shaping techniques.

Key Word

A **key word** is a word in which the client successfully produces the treatment target. Although any word can be a key word, many times key words have special significance for a client, such as the name of a favorite toy or person. Treatment based on a key word seeks to generalize success in producing the sound to other words and phonetic environments.

Phonetic Placement and Shaping

Phonetic placement involves the physical placement of a client's articulators into position to produce a sound. Phonetic placement of [t], for example, entails giving detailed instructions that guide the client to quickly touch the alveolar ridge with the tongue tip. **Shaping** is developing a new sound from a sound already in the client's phonetic inventory. Shaping techniques, for example, provide a series of steps through which [t] might be shaped into [s]. Treatment seeks to generalize success in performing phonetic placement and shaping techniques to spontaneous speech.

MOST AND LEAST KNOWLEDGE METHODS

Most often, treatment targets require a client to acquire new sounds and syllables. There are two methods to determine how similar treatment targets should be compared to the client's current articulation and phonological abilities: the most knowledge method and the least knowledge method.

Most Knowledge Method

The **most knowledge method** is a traditional criterion to choose treatment targets. In this method, treatment targets differ minimally from the sounds that the client already produces (Elbert & Gierut, 1986). This is based on the client having a great deal of knowledge about the treatment target, because he or she is producing many features of the treatment target in other sounds. For example, within the most knowledge method the treatment target for a client whose phonetic inventory contained one oral stop ([p]) and no fricatives would likely be another oral stop—perhaps a sound that differed only in voicing (i.e., [b]) or in place of production (i.e., [t] or [k]). The close similarity between the client's existing abilities and the treatment target is intended to ensure that the new sound will be acquired without great frustration for the client (Van Riper, 1978). A possible limitation of a most knowledge method is that treatment must proceed in small increments, which is time consuming with clients who have multiple articulation and phonological errors. To acquire the entire set of oral stops, for example, the above client's treatment targets would include [b], [t], [d], [k], and [g].

Least Knowledge Method

In a **least knowledge method**, treatment targets differ from the client's existing abilities by multiple features (Elbert & Gierut, 1986; Powell, 1991). The client just described whose speech contained one oral stop ([p]) and no fricatives, for example, might have [z] as a treatment target. The essential idea underlying a least knowledge method is that treatment targets should afford the client the opportunity to acquire skills needed to produce more than single sounds. In acquiring [z], for example, the client also acquires a new contrast in place of production (bilabial and alveolar), a new voicing contrast (voiceless and voiced), and a new manner of production (stop and fricative). Presently, the least knowledge method is a relatively new proposal and its effectiveness has been studied only with a small number of subjects. The results of these investigations appear promising for the least knowledge method as an alternative to the more traditional most knowledge method for clients whose speech contains multiple errors.

NUMBER OF TREATMENT TARGETS

Typically, only one treatment target is facilitated per session. This is because many clients find it confusing to receive treatment on more than one treatment target in a single session. An exception to this general rule is made for clients requiring a flexible approach (see next section) or when a clinician chooses a multiple phoneme approach.

Concurrent treatment targets can be facilitated for weeks or months. Two general strategies are used to help decide how many treatment targets to facilitate simultaneously: training deep and training wide (Elbert & Gierut, 1986). **Training deep** provides intensive treatment on one or two treatment targets, which allows proportionally more attention to be devoted to each treatment target than is the case when a greater number of treatment targets are employed.

Training wide provides treatment on three or more treatment targets, which offers the client more opportunities to discover relationships between targets than if a training deep strategy is selected. A client who receives treatment on [p], [d], and [s], for example, is being exposed to contrasts in place of production (bilabial and alveolar), voicing (voiced and voiceless), and manner (stop and fricative).

CHANGING TREATMENT TARGETS

An important consideration is determining when to change from one treatment target to another during the course of treatment. In this book, the three criteria for changing treatment targets are flexibility, time, and percentage.

Flexibility

If a **flexible criterion** is used, a treatment target is facilitated until the client becomes disinterested, at which point another treatment target is facilitated. An illustration of a flexible criterion is the statement: "Treatment for [b] will continue for as long as the client's interest is sustained."

Time

If a **time criterion** is used, a certain amount of treatment time (typically, 60 minutes) is devoted to each target (Hodson, 1989). After the time has elapsed, treatment shifts to another treatment target. After treatment for all targets is met (called **a cycle**), the treatment targets are treated again (a second cycle). Cycles are repeated until all treatment targets are remediated, which typically requires from three to four cycles (approximately 1 year of treatment). An illustration of a time criterion is the statement, "Treatment for [t] will be provided for 1 hour in cycle 1."

Percentage

If a **percentage criterion** is used, a treatment target is facilitated until a certain percentage correct is reached. An illustration of a percentage criterion is the statement: "Correct production of [s] in word initial position 75% of the time."

LINGUISTIC LEVEL AND PHONETIC ENVIRONMENTS

Treatment targets typically are introduced in a single linguistic level in either one or two phonetic environments. The possible linguistic levels are isolated sounds, nonsense syllables, words, phrases, sentences, and spontaneous speech; the possible phonetic environments are word positions (initial, medial, final) and syllable positions (syllable initial, final, intervocalic, stressed and unstressed syllable, etc.). The most likely phonetic environments in which to introduce treatment targets are listed in Table 15–2 (Bleile, 1991). However, as with most clinical enterprises, the clinician does best to follow the client's lead in selecting both the number and types of phonetic environments in which to introduce treatment targets. If, for example, the client is more successful producing velar stops between vowels, then treatment should begin by facilitating velar stops in that position. Similarly, if the client appears stimulable for [t] in both word-initial and word-final positions, the clinician may consider beginning treatment in both positions.

Exercise 15–1: Treatment Targets

Long-term goals, short-term goals, and treatment targets are each important concepts in articulation and phonological treatment. This exercise focuses on the distinction between goals and treatment targets.

QUESTIONS

1. How do treatment targets differ from long-term goals?

2. How do treatment targets differ from short-term goals?

3. Describe a long-term goal, short-term goals, and treatment targets for a client 20 months of age who was born 3 months premature. Nearly 80% of the words in the client's expressive vocabulary are pronounced as [bi]. The clinician elects to use flooding to reduce the number of homonyms.

4. Describe a long-term goal, short-term goals, and treatment targets for a client 4 years of age whose cognitive development approximates that of a child 2 years, 6 months of age. The most prominent error patterns in the client's speech are Fronting, Gliding, and Stopping. The clinician selects to work on [k] to eliminate Fronting and on [f] to begin to eliminate Stopping. The client elects not to work on sounds affected by Gliding at this time.

5. Describe a long-term goal, short-term goals, and treatment targets for a client 7 years of age who says [w] for [r]. The client has no intellectual or cognitive impairments and is not teased about speech.

TABLE 15–2. "Best bets" for environments within which to establish treatment targets.

Treatment Targets	Environments
All treatment targets	Establish in CV, CVCV, or VC syllables
All treatment targets	Establish in stressed syllables
Consonants	Except for the instances noted below, establish consonants in the beginning of words
Voiced consonants	Establish either between vowels or in the beginning of words and syllables
Voiceless consonants	Establish at the end of syllables and words
Velar stops	Establish at the end of words or at the beginning of words before a back vowel
Alveolar stops	Establish at the beginning of words before front vowels
Voiced fricatives	Establish between vowels

From *Child Phonology: A Book of Exercises for Students* (p. 78), by K. Bleile, 1991, San Diego: Singular Publishing Group. Copyright by Singular Publishing Group. Reprinted with permission.

Answer Sheet for Exercise 15–1: Treatment Targets

1. **Long-term goals and treatment targets:**

2. **Short-term goals and treatment targets:**

3. **Long-term goal:**
   Short-term goal:
   Treatment target:

4. **Long-term goal:**
   Short-term goals:
   Treatment targets:

5. **Long-term goal:**
   Short-term goals:
   Treatment target:

Exercise 15–2: Treatment Targets

This exercise asks you to describe which statement best corresponds to a treatment target option.

QUESTIONS

1. A treatment target is facilitated until the client becomes disinterested. *This is an example and is answered for you.*

2. A treatment target differs minimally from the sounds the client already produces.

3. A sound is selected for treatment because it is produced correctly on 10% to 49% of all occasions in one or more phonetic environments.

4. Intensive treatment is provided to one or two treatment targets.

5. A certain amount of time is devoted to each treatment target.

6. A sound is selected for treatment because it is produced correctly in one or a few words.

7. A treatment target differs from the client's existing abilities by multiple features.

8. A sound is selected for treatment because it can be imitated correctly.

9. Treatment is provided for three or more treatment targets.

10. A treatment target is facilitated until a percentage of correct productions is obtained.

11. A sound is selected for treatment because it can be produced correctly either through physical placement or can be developed from a sound already in the client's phonetic inventory.

Answer Sheet for Exercise 15–2: Treatment Targets

1. **Technique:** flexibility

2. **Technique:**

3. **Technique:**

4. **Technique:**

5. **Technique:**

6. **Technique:**

7. **Technique:**

8. **Technique:**

9. **Technique:**

10. **Technique:**

11. **Technique:**

Exercise 15–3: Treatment Targets

The least knowledge method is a new addition to the clinical armamentarium. Because it offers the promise of promoting generalization (and thus speed the treatment process), it is an important concept to master for those who treat clients experiencing difficulties with entire sound classes. The present exercise illustrates differences between using most and least knowledge methods to select treatment targets. The speech sample on which the exercise is based is from E, the child whose tracheostomy was removed when she was 2 years, 4 months of age (Bleile, Stark, & Silverman McGowan, 1993). The following words are E's entire expressive vocabulary 6 weeks after decannulation.

Least Knowledge Method

The investigators who proposed the least knowledge method recommend its use regardless of stimulability (Elbert & Gierut, 1986; Powell, 1991). The reason for this is that the investigators believe that sounds for which a client is stimulable are likely to improve without treatment. The investigators note that treatment proceeds somewhat slower if stimulability is not used, but that treatment gains offset this additional time. My suggestion to the reader is to try the investigators' approach to determine if it is successful for you. My clinical experience is that a client generally has great frustration with treatment targets for which he or she demonstrates no production capacity, especially if the client has concomitant cognitive or attention limitations. I also have found extensive individual differences in the prognosis of stimulable sounds—some clients appearing to need treatment to acquire sounds for which they are stimulable and others improving on such sounds spontaneously. An important area of research is to determine the prognosis for sounds for which a client shows some production capacity, whether produced through stimulability or emerging, in key words or phonetic environments, or through phonetic placement and shaping techniques.

SPEECH SAMPLE

Intended Words	E
1. bottle	baba
2. bubble	baba
3. Pop Pop*	dada
4. daddy	dada
5. mom	mam
6. up	ʌp

* = Pop Pop is the family name for grandfather

QUESTIONS

1. The most and least knowledge methods offer the greatest contrast in selecting treatment targets for clients like E who have difficulty with entire classes of sounds. For this illustration, suppose E is stimulable for word initial [p] and [k]. Which sound do you select as a treatment target using a most knowledge method? Why?

2. Which sound ([p] or [k]) do you select using a least knowledge method?

3. To further illustrate possible differences between the most and least knowledge method, suppose that E is stimulable for [t] and [s] rather than [p] and [k]. Which sound do you select using a most knowledge method?

4. Which sound ([t] or [s]) do you select using a least knowledge method?

5. Lastly, as further practice, suppose that E is stimulable for [f] and [s] rather than [t] and [s]. Which sound do you select using a most knowledge method?

6. Which sound ([s] or [f]) do you select using a least knowledge method?

7. *For discussion:* If a least knowledge method is used, which sound do you select if they differ by the same number of distinctive features? For example, suppose that E is stimulable for [t] and [g] rather than the sounds presented above. In this situation, do you select [t] (which differs in voicing from the other sounds) or [g] (which differs in place of production)?

Answer Sheet for Exercise 15–3: Treatment Targets

1. **Most knowledge method:**

2. **Least knowledge method:**

3. **Most knowledge method:**

4. **Least knowledge method:**

5. **Most knowledge method:**

6. **Least knowledge method:**

7. *For discussion:*

Exercise 15–4: Treatment Targets

For each client the clinician must select treatment targets, decide between most and least knowledge methods, determine the number of treatment targets, decide how to change treatment targets, and select the linguistic level and phonetic environments within which to facilitate treatment targets.

This exercise focuses on treatment decisions that arise in the care of Gavin, the client in stage 2 whose long- and short-term goals were discussed in the previous chapter. Assume for this exercise that Gavin's short-term goal is to reduce variability in specific words.

SPEECH SAMPLE

See Appendix C–3.

QUESTIONS

1. An important step in seeking to reduce variability is to identify key words in which one or more sounds is produced correctly. Which of Gavin's words contain a sound or sounds produced correctly? *This is an example and is answered for you.*

2. Identify the potential treatment targets in Gavin's key words.

3. Gavin's potential treatment targets offer many opportunities to select between most and least knowledge methods. Which option (most or least knowledge method) do you select? Why?

4. Suppose you select a most knowledge method and training deep. Which two treatment targets do you select? Why? (**Hint:** For this and the following question there is more than one "correct" pair of sounds you might select.)

5. Instead of a most knowledge method and training deep, suppose you select a least knowledge method and training wide. List two consonant treatment targets you might select. Explain your choices.

6. Treatment also involves deciding between options for changing from one treatment target to another. Most clinicians would likely consider a percentage criterion the least viable option for Gavin. Why?

7. Which option to change treatment targets do you select for Gavin? Why?

8. Treatment also requires deciding at which linguistic level and phonetic environments to begin treatment. Most clinicians would likely consider both the isolated sound and the phrase level to be poor options for Gavin. Why?

9. What linguistic level do you select for Gavin? Why?

10. What is the phonetic environment (in terms of syllable structure) of the treatment targets in Gavin's key words?

Answer Sheet for Exercise 15–4: Treatment Targets

1. **Words:** *pig, cat, door, fish, fan, cheese, house,* and *rabbit*

2. **Treatment targets:**

3. **Most or least knowledge:**

4. **Most knowledge and training deep:**

5. **Least knowledge and training wide:**

6. **Changing treatment targets (percentage):**

7. **Changing treatment targets:**

8. **Linguistic level (isolated sound or phrase):**

9. **Linguistic level:**

10. **Phonetic environment:**

Exercise 15–5: Treatment Targets

This exercise considers treatment decisions that arise in the care of Kelly, the client in stage 3 whose long- and short-term goals were discussed in the previous chapter. For this exercise assume that Kelly's short-term goal is to eliminate errors affecting sound classes. Assume also that an error pattern approach is used, and that the error patterns selected for treatment are Stopping, Gliding, Cluster Reduction, and Affrication.

SPEECH SAMPLE

See Appendix C–7.

QUESTIONS

1. Many times possible treatment targets are selected based on a combination of factors, including the speech sample, stimulability testing, the results of word probes, and the findings of trials of phonetic placement and shaping. However, for this exercise identify possible treatment targets based solely on the speech sample in Appendix C–7. Focus first on Stopping. To identify possible treatment targets for this error pattern, identify any words in the speech sample in which fricatives (a sound class often affected by Stopping) are produced correctly. (**Hint:** First identify which sounds typically undergo this error pattern. Next, determine if these sounds are produced correctly in any words in the speech sample. Such sounds are potential treatment targets because Kelly demonstrates a capacity to produce them on at least some occasions.) *This is an example and is answered for you.*

2. Follow the same procedure as in the first question to select which sounds in the speech sample are possible treatment targets for Gliding, Cluster Reduction, and Affrication.

3. Summarize your list of possible treatment target for each error pattern. *The first part of this question is an example and is answered for you.*

4. You also need to decide how similar the treatment targets should be compared to Kelly's current articulation and phonological abilities (most knowledge method or least knowledge method). Which option (most or least knowledge method) do you select? Why?

5. Which option (training wide or training deep) do you select? Why?

6. Another clinical decision to make concerns when to change from one treatment target to another. Which option do you select? Why?

7. Which linguistic level or levels do you select? Why?

8. Lastly, you need to consider the phonetic environments within which to begin treatment. Based on Kelly's speech sample, which phonetic environments do you select? (*Hint:* Use the words you identified in the second question to answer this question.) *The first part of the question is an example and is answered for you.*

Answer Sheet for Exercise 15–5: Treatment Targets

1. **Possible treatment targets:**
   Stopping: [z] (zoo)
                [v] (van, vest)

2. **Possible treatment targets:**
   Gliding:
   Cluster Reduction:
   Affrication:

3. **Summary of possible treatment targets:**
   Stopping: [z v]
   Gliding:
   Cluster Reduction:
   Affrication:

4. **Most or least knowledge:**

5. **Training wide or deep:**

6. **Changing treatment targets:**

7. **Linguistic level:**

8. **Phonetic environments:**
   Stopping: [z] word finally
   　　　　　　[v] word initially
   Gliding: [l]
   　　　　　　[r]
   Cluster Reduction: [tʃr]
   　　　　　　　　　　　[kl]
   　　　　　　　　　　　nasal + stop
   Affrication: [s]

Exercise 15–6: Treatment Targets

This exercise considers treatment decisions that arise in the care of Billy, the client in Stage 4 whose long- and short-term goals were discussed in the previous chapter. Assume for this exercise that Billy's short-term goal is elimination of errors affecting word initial [r] outside of consonant clusters, and that results of a word probe indicate that Billy is stimulable for the short-term goal approximately 30% of the time (see Exercise 11–6 for a discussion of the word probe).

SPEECH SAMPLE

See Appendix C–8.

QUESTIONS

1. Suppose you ask Billy to lie on his back on the floor, to relax his mouth, and to say "rrr." What technique are you using to help select a treatment target?

2. You need to decide whether to use a most or least knowledge method to select treatment targets. Which method do you select? Why?

3. Which option do you select—to train wide or to train deep? Why?

4. Which option do you select to decide when to change from one treatment target to another—flexibility, time, or percentage? Why?

5. At which linguistic level or levels do you select to begin treatment? Why?

6. What word position do you select to begin treatment? Does the phonetic environment include specific vowels? Why or why not? (*Hint:* See Exercise 8–6 to help answer the question about vowel context.)

Answer Sheet for Exercise 15–6: Treatment Targets

1. **Selection technique:**

2. **Most or least knowledge:**

3. **Training deep or wide:**

4. **Changing treatment targets:**

5. **Linguistic level:**

6. **Phonetic environment:**

CHAPTER
16

Administrative Decisions

Treatment requires the clinician to make administrative decisions about the organization of treatment sessions, including whether to provide treatment individually or in groups, the frequency and length of sessions, length of individual treatment activities, and format of activities.

TYPES OF SESSIONS

Treatment can be provided in either individual or group sessions. Individual sessions consist of a single client and are often preferred during the early stages of treatment when the clinician is introducing new treatment targets. Group sessions typically consist of three to five clients of roughly similar ages and developmental levels and are often preferred in the middle and late stages of therapy, when goals shift from introducing new treatment targets to helping clients to generalize and maintain what has been learned.

FREQUENCY OF SESSIONS

Treatment for clients at all levels of articulation and phonological development typically is provided

---

Inclusion

Inclusion is the provision of speech and language treatment within classroom settings. Inclusion is an old idea that has recently regained popularity. The reasons for the resurgence in interest in inclusion are both educational and financial. The primary educational reason is the desire among many parents and educators to include persons with disabilities in as non-restrictive a setting as possible. Financially, inclusion often costs school districts much less than providing individual care. Most educators do not consider inclusion an exclusive choice, and they provide inclusion, individual care, and group sessions in conjunction with each other. When a good relationship exists between the speech-language pathologist and the classroom teacher, inclusion provides an extremely important way to help a client to practice and generalize the results of treatment.

from two to five times a week. Some evidence exists that intensive therapy four to five times a week is slightly more efficient for clients in Stage 4 than less intensive therapy of twice a week for a longer number of weeks (Bernthal & Bankson, 1993).

LENGTH OF SESSIONS

Individual therapy sessions range from 10 to 15 minutes to 1 hour. Group sessions typically range from 30 to 45 minutes.

LENGTH OF ACTIVITIES IN SESSIONS

Individual activities in sessions may last from less than a minute to nearly 30 minutes.

FORMAT OF ACTIVITIES

There are four basic types of activities: drill, drill play, structured play, and play (Shriberg & Kwiatkowski, 1982). **Drill** involves the clinician presenting material for mass practice by the client in such activities as repeating lists of words, naming pictures, and so on. **Drill play** involves drills presented in the context of games such as spinning wheels, game boards, and so on. **Structured play** is drill play presented through play-like activities such as playing house, shopping, parking toy cars in a garage, and so on. **Play** is defined as child-oriented activities during which acquisition of targets is facilitated during the course of the activities.

Exercise 16–1: Administrative Decisions

This exercise offers a chance to address questions about administrative decisions that arise in the care of clients with articulation and phonological disorders.

QUESTIONS

1. Why are individual sessions often preferred during the early phases of treatment? Why are group sessions often preferred during the middle and late phases of treatment?

2. Why do you suppose that for Stage 4 clients intensive treatment sessions 4 to 5 times weekly is somewhat more effective than treatment sessions 2 times weekly over a longer period of time?

3. What is the typical range of length of sessions and length of activities in sessions?

4. What are the options for format of activities?

Answer Sheet for Exercise 16–1: Administrative Decisions

1. **Sessions:**

2. **Session frequency:**

3. **Length of sessions:**
   Length of activities in sessions:

4. **Formats:**

Exercise 16–2: Administrative Decisions

The care of each client involves making a number of administrative decisions. This and the following two exercises consider the administrative decisions that arise in the care of Gavin, Kelly, and Billy. The present exercise focuses on Gavin, the client in Stage 2 whose goals and treatment targets were discussed in previous chapters.

SPEECH SAMPLE

See Appendix C–3.

QUESTIONS

1. What type of treatment session do you select?

2. What frequency of treatment do you select?

3. What length of treatment sessions do you select?

4. What length of activities within sessions do you select?

5. What format of activities do you select?

Answer Sheet for Exercise 16–2: Administrative Decisions

1. **Type of sessions:**

2. **Frequency of sessions:**

3. **Length of sessions:**

4. **Length of activities:**

5. **Format of activities:**

Exercise 16–3: Administrative Decisions

This exercise focuses on Kelly, the client in Stage 3 whose goals and treatment targets were discussed in previous chapters.

SPEECH SAMPLE

See Appendix C–7.

QUESTIONS

1. What type of treatment session do you select?
2. What frequency of treatment do you select?
3. What length of treatment sessions do you select?
4. What length of activities within sessions do you select?
5. What format of activities do you select?

Answer Sheet for Exercise 16–3: Administrative Decisions

1. **Type of sessions:**

2. **Frequency of sessions:**

3. **Length of sessions:**

4. **Length of activities:**

5. **Format of activities:**

Exercise 16–4: Administrative Decisions

This exercise focuses on Billy, the client in Stage 4 whose goals and treatment targets were discussed in previous chapters.

SPEECH SAMPLE

See Appendix C–8.

QUESTIONS

1. What type of treatment session do you select?

2. What frequency of treatment do you select?

3. What length of treatment sessions do you select?

4. What length of activities within sessions do you select?

5. What format of activities do you select?

Answer Sheet for Exercise 16–4: Administrative Decisions

1. **Type of sessions:**

2. **Frequency of sessions:**

3. **Length of sessions:**

4. **Length of activities:**

5. **Format of activities:**

CHAPTER
17

Assessing Treatment Progress

Assessing the effectiveness of treatment is essential to care provision for all clients, not least because periodic assessments of progress are required by law, by most workplaces, and for reimbursement by insurance companies. The need for information on treatment outcome was listed as the highest health care priority by a recent American Speech-Language-Hearing Association task force (Task Force on Health Care, 1993). The two major options to assess treatment progress are pre- and posttests and ongoing information gathering.

PRE- AND POSTTESTS

As the names suggest, **pretests** are administered prior to treatment (often as part of the assessment) and **posttests** are administered at major junctures in treatment, often to determine if short- or long-term goals have been attained. Many clinicians, myself included, prefer pre- and posttests to assess treatment progress because they are quick and easy to administer and do not take attention away from a client during treatment sessions.

How Much Progress Is Needed to Make a Difference?

Most methods to assess treatment progress only indicate if a behavior occurs more or less often than at a given previous time. Yet, for some clients an improvement of a few percentage points might cause a clinician to celebrate, although for another client the clinician might not be satisfied with anything less than perfect performance. For this reason, a percentage cannot represent whether treatment progress has been sufficient to make a difference. Such a judgment is made based on clinical experience and, whenever possible, through consultation with the client and important people in the client's life. Measures of functional outcome such as client satisfaction surveys and reduction in the need for future clinical services are two of many ways to determine if treatment has improved the client's life.

Two quick and effective types of pre- and posttests are word probes and judgment scales of severity and/or intelligibility. Many times a client receives both types of pre- and posttests.

Word probes can easily be adapted into pre- and posttests for clients in Stages 3 or 4. To illustrate, a sound probe might indicate that a client was able to produce [s] 2 of 5 times word initially and none of 5 times between vowels and word finally. This information could be used as the pretest, and the probe could be given again at the completion of treatment as the posttest. (There is no "correct" number of words that should be included in a probe. A general rule of thumb is ten words per treatment target). Error probes also can be used as pre- and posttests. To illustrate, the client might demonstrate a Fronting pattern on 8 of 10 words (80%) during the pretest and might demonstrate Fronting on 2 of 10 words (20%) on the posttest.

Judgment scales of severity and intelligibility often serve as pre- and posttests to assess treatment progress. If the judges are clinicians, three clinicians should be used, if possible. A problem with clinical judgments of severity and intelligibility is that the faster types are highly subjective. Also, measures that show only a few degrees of disability may not be sufficiently sensitive to detect smaller increments of improvement. Results of intelligibility and severity judgment scales might be reported as, "Three of three trained speech-language clinicians judged the client to have a severe speech disorder before the onset of therapy. The client is now judged to have a mild speech disorder."

ONGOING INFORMATION GATHERING

Although more time consuming than performing pre- and posttests, some clinicians collect ongoing information on a client's progress toward meeting a therapy objective. During each treatment session, for example, the clinician tabulates the client's rate of success, usually as a percentage value. To illustrate, the clinician might tabulate that the client is 50% accurate in producing a treatment target during session 1, 58% accurate in session 2, 64% accurate in session 3, and so on. Ongoing information gathering has the important advantage over pre- and posttesting in that it allows the clinician to monitor the client's treatment progress more closely.

Single-subject design experiments offer a more rigorous type of ongoing information gathering. Single-subject design experiments provide a method to demonstrate that improvement in a client results from the clinician's treatment, rather than from extraneous factors such as time and maturation. Although commonly employed in behavioral psychology, single-subject design experiments have not found their way into widespread clinical use in speech-language pathology. Perhaps this is because the experiments are time-consuming to perform and their use requires some specialized knowledge. The information below outlines the basic steps and logic behind one type of single-subject design experiment, called a multiple baseline design. Before attempting such an experiment, the reader is referred to the more complete discussions on this topic appearing in McReynolds and Kearns (1983).

The type of single-subject design experiment that is most applicable to the clinical care of articulation and phonological disorders is called a **multiple baseline design**. A multiple baseline design can be used to evaluate treatment if (1) the client has at least two potential treatment targets and (2) the client's treatment targets are not so closely related that, when the clinician treats one target, the other target will also improve. For example, [p] and [b] would probably not be suitable treatment targets in a single-subject design experiment, because in many cases when a clinician focuses on [p] (or [b]) the cognate also improves. Better treatment targets for a single-subject design experiment might be [p] and [s], because improving one would not be expected to improve the other.

Multiple baseline design experiments consist of two phases, called A (**baseline**) and B (**treatment**). During the baseline no treatment on the treatment target is provided. The baseline and treatment phases each must be at least three intervals (usually treatment sessions) in length. To illustrate, data are collected during baseline for at least three treatment sessions, and treatment is provided for at least the same (and most likely longer) number of sessions. Changes in percentage values between the baseline and treatment phases are the means most frequently used to demonstrate treatment progress. The results of the experiment are usually displayed as a simple graph of the type shown in Figure 17–1.

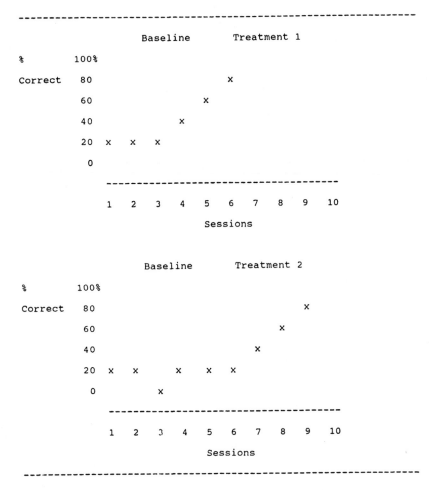

Figure 17–1. Example of a multiple baseline experiment.

Exercise 17–1: Assessing Treatment Progress

This exercise reviews the basic options to assess treatment progress.

QUESTIONS

1. Identify two types of pre- and posttests.
2. When developing a word probe for pre- and posttesting, what is the general rule for how many words to include per each treatment target?
3. What are advantages of using judgment scales of severity and/or intelligibility as pre- and posttests?
4. What are disadvantages in using judgment scales of severity and/or intelligibility as pre- and posttests?
5. What is an advantage of ongoing information gathering over pre- and posttesting?
6. What is a disadvantage of ongoing information gathering compared to pre- and posttesting?
7. What's the major difference between single subject design experiments and methods to assess treatment progress such as pre- and posttests and daily information gathering?

8. Why are [t] and [d] not good treatment targets to include as the across behaviors in a multiple baseline single-subject design experiment?

9. *For discussion:* Standardized articulation and phonological assessment instruments are sometimes used as pre- and posttests. These often fail to show treatment progress, even when the clinician can easily demonstrate progress through a variety of other means. Why do you suppose standardized assessment instruments often are not sensitive to therapeutic gains?

Answer Sheet for Exercise 17–1: Assessing Treatment Progress

1. **Pre- and posttests:**

2. **Number of words:**

3. **Advantages:**

4. **Disadvantages:**

5. **Advantage:**

6. **Disadvantage:**

7. **Difference:**

8. **[t] and [d]:**

9. *For discussion:*

Exercise 17–2: Assessing Treatment Progress

This exercise considers ways to assess the treatment progress of Tommy, the 5-year-old child with Down syndrome whose speech was analyzed in Exercise 14–3 (Bodine, 1974).

SPEECH SAMPLE

Intended Words	Tommy
1. piece	bi
2. please	bi
3. B	bi
4. big	bi
5. talk	da
6. Kathy	da
7. coffee	da
8. Jack	da
9. jacket	da
10. that	da
11. chocolate	da

QUESTIONS

1. Suppose you select reduction in homonyms as a short-term goal for Tommy and decide to accomplish this through eliminating Prevocalic Voicing. The treatment targets are [p t k tʃ] (the sounds affected by Prevocalic Voicing). What are your options for pre-tests to determine the frequency with which Prevocalic Voicing occurs?

2. Suppose you elect to use the 11-word speech sample as a pretest. What is the percentage of occurrence of Prevocalic Voicing in Tommy's speech prior to treatment?

3. Suppose you decide to use ongoing information gathering to assess treatment progress. How often do you assess Tommy's therapeutic gains?

4. Suppose you decide to use pre- and posttests to assess treatment progress. How often do you assess Tommy's therapeutic gains?

5. Suppose treatment for Prevocalic Voicing is nearing completion and you decide to administer a posttest (if you utilize ongoing information gathering, the posttest is the last session in which information is tabulated). How do you develop a posttest to determine the frequency with which Prevocalic Voicing occurs?

6. Suppose the posttest indicates that Prevocalic Voicing occurs 25% of all possible occurrences. Does this prove that Tommy's treatment is effective? Why or why not?

7. What method to assess treatment progress might you use to know with greater certainty that Tommy's improvement is the result of treatment?

Answer Sheet for Exercise 17–2: Assessing Treatment Progress

1. **Pretest:**

2. **Pretest:**

3. **Ongoing information gathering:**

4. **Pre- and posttests:**

5. **Posttest:**

6. **Treatment effect:**

7. **Assessment method:**

Exercise 17–3: Assessing Treatment Progress

This exercise focuses on assessing the treatment progress of Gavin, the client in Stage 2 who was discussed in exercises in previous chapters. Assume for this exercise that Gavin's short-term goal is to reduce variability in specific words.

SPEECH SAMPLE

See Appendix C–3.

QUESTIONS

1. How could you use Gavin's speech sample as a pretest for his short-term goal?

2. What is the extent of interword variability in Gavin's speech sample?

3. Suppose treatment is nearing completion and you decide to administer a posttest. Should the words on the posttest be those that received treatment? Or should different words be included in the posttest? Why or why not?

4. *For discussion:* When should the words being treated be included in the pre- and posttests?

5. *For discussion:* When should the words being treated not be included on the pre- and posttests?

Answer Sheet for Exercise 17–3: Assessing Treatment Progress

1. **Pretest:**

2. **Variability:**

3. **Posttest:**

4. *For discussion:*

5. *For discussion:*

Exercise 17–4: Assessing Treatment Progress

This exercise focuses on assessing the treatment progress of Kelly, the client in Stage 3 who was discussed in exercises in previous chapters. Assume for this exercise that Kelly's short-term goal is elimination of errors affecting sound classes, and that the error patterns selected for treatment are Stopping, Gliding, Cluster Reduction, and Affrication.

SPEECH SAMPLE

See Appendix C–7.

QUESTIONS

1. Describe the major options for pretests to assess Kelly's treatment progress.
2. Suppose you select word probes for pretests. Develop a five-word error probe to assess the occurrence of Stopping in word initial position. (*Hint:* Kelly's dialect does not include the interdental fricatives, so you need not include those sounds in your probes.)
3. Develop another five-word probe to assess Cluster Reduction in word initial position.
4. Do you provide treatment to the same words included on the pre- and posttests?
5. *For discussion:* When should five-word probes be used? When 10 words? When should error probes assess error patterns in all word positions? When only in one or two positions?

Answer Sheet for Exercise 17–4: Assessing Treatment Progress

1. **Options:**

2. **Error probe:**

3. **Error probe:**

4. **Treatment:**

5. *For discussion:*

Exercise 17–5: Assessing Treatment Progress

This exercise focuses on assessing the treatment progress of Billy, the client in Stage 4 who was discussed in exercises in Chapters 14, 15, and 16. Assume for this exercise that Billy's short-term goal is to eliminate errors affecting word initial [r] outside of consonant clusters, and that results of a word probe indicate that Billy is stimulable for the short-term goal approximately 30% of the time.

SPEECH SAMPLE

See Appendix C–8.

QUESTIONS

1. Can you use the results of a word probe for stimulability testing as a pretest? Why or why not?

2. How might you state the results of the word probe in a clinical report?

3. If the word probe is used as a pretest, does the posttest need to obtained using imitation? Why or why not?

4. Suppose posttest results are obtained using imitation, and that the results of the posttest indicates Billy pronounces [r] correctly 70% of the time. Can you know with certainty that the change between the pre- and posttest is the result of treatment?

Answer Sheet for Exercise 17–5: Assessing Treatment Progress

1. **Imitation:**

2. **Clinical report:**

3. **Posttest:**

4. **Treatment result:**

SECTION
V

Facilitative Techniques

with Patricia Dukes

OVERVIEW

Methods to change a client's articulation and phonological development are called **facilitative techniques**. The term "facilitative" is usually preferred to "teaching" or "instruction" to emphasize that treatment is an interaction between the clinician's efforts and the client's capacity and willingness to learn. The chapters in this section describe facilitative techniques for bombardment, increasing awareness, facilitating syllables and words, and indirect and direct techniques. (**Hint:** Some students cut out the activities described in the answer sheet and file them on 3 × 5 inch cards.)

Andy Warhol Was Right

Andy Warhol predicted that in the future everyone would be famous for 15 minutes. The future already is here for children's heros and villains. In the blink of an eye (or so it seems) Luke Skywalker and Darth Vader have given way to Ninja Turtles, who in turn have been supplanted in children's affections by Batman, Pocahontas, and the Mighty Morphin Power Rangers. Because fame is so fleeting among children, the specific names of heros and villains appearing in activities in this section are generally left unspecified. You or the client should fill in names with whomever is popular at the moment.

CHAPTER
18

Bombardment

Children typically acquire the sounds and syllables they hear most often. Bombardment is a well-established method used to increase the relative frequency of a treatment target in the client's environment (Nemoy & Davis, 1954). Typically, a client is not required to speak or vocalize during bombardment activities—only to listen. Some clinicians also recommend that the client wear a frequency modulated (FM) system during bombardment activities to further increase the treatment target's saliency (Hodson, 1989). Depending on the client's age and the clinician's treatment philosophy, bombardment activities may last from a few to 10 minutes. Some clinicians undertake bombardment only when introducing a new treatment target. Other clinicians include bombardment activities as part of each treatment session.

Scripting

Students inexperienced with bombardment techniques may wish to script their verbalizations ahead of time for the first few treatment sessions so that opportunities for bombardment are maximized. To illustrate, a possible script for a bombardment activity for [f] based on a stuffed bear might begin, "I'd like you to meet my friend. His name is Polar. He is a bear. He is not a real bear. He is a teddy bear. Polar feels furry. Do you have a teddy bear?"

Exercise 18–1: Bombardment

Bombardment is used to increase the frequency of treatment targets in the client's environment. This exercise is based on the speech of Ethan, a child 1 year, 8 months of age who was born 2 months pre-maturely through induced labor because, as Ethan's mother reports, "the fetus had stopped growing in utero" (Lee, 1994).

SPEECH SAMPLE

Intended Words	Ethan
1. balloon	b̪ʌwʊ
2. banana	b̪ʌ
3. bus	b̪ʌ
4. duck	dæɸ
5. dog	gɔ
6. down	dʌm
7. cake	te
8. car	dʌ
9. cookie	tuʔi
10. kite	haɪ
10. sock	tʌ
11. sun	tʌ
12. nose	noʊ
13. eat	di
14. apple	ʌb̪ʌ
15. up	ʌb̪
16. in	ʌɸ
17. ?	əgʌ
18. ?	ʌm
19. ?	hʌhoʊ
20. ?	hʌm
21. ?	tɪb̪ʊ
22. ?	kʌhoʊ
23. ?	gʌʔ
24. ?	nʌ
25. ?	gæ
26. ?	tʌ
27. ?	gʌdɪ
28. ?	hæm
29. ?	tɪ

QUESTIONS

1. Ethan's speech is notable for a lack of fricatives, the exception being a word final voiceless bilabial fricative in *duck* (fourth word). Suppose that Ethan's clinician chooses word initial [f] as a treatment target. Develop a "reading" activity about fish in which to bombard Ethan with [f]. (**Hint:** Give examples of some specific words you would use.) *This question is an example and is answered for you.*

2. Suppose that Ethan displays no interest in the fish subject, but instead wants to see pictures in his favorite book about babies. Adapt the book Ethan selects into a bombardment activity for [f].

3. Interactive games provide another opportunity for bombardment activities. Develop a bombardment activity for [f] based on playing with toy cars and a toy parking garage.

4. For additional practice, develop another bombardment activity for [f] that relies on interactive play.

5. Activities for daily living (ADLs) involve other opportunities for bombardment activities. Develop a bombardment activity for [f] based on eating a snack.

6. For additional practice, develop another bombardment activity for [f] based on an ADL.

7. *For discussion:* Bombardment typically is part of a treatment package that also includes production. However, a clinician might elect to provide bombardment without attempting to facilitate production if the client appears stalled in articulation and phonological development. Why might a clinician provide bombardment in such a circumstance? Do you think bombardment is effective without also facilitating production?

Answer Sheet for Exercise 18–1: Bombardment

1. **Fish book:** Present Ethan with a large brightly colored picture book about fish. Show Ethan pictures in the book, highlighting words containing [f], such as *fish*, *fins*, *fly* (for catching fish), *fishing boots*, and *fire* (for cooking fish).

2. **Baby book:**

3. **Cars and garage:**

4. **Interactive play:**

5. **Snack:**

6. **ADL:**

7. *For discussion:*

Exercise 18–2: Bombardment

This exercise focuses on developing bombardment activities for Tess. Tess is 4 years, 4 months of age and is mildly delayed in both Korean and English, the two languages to which she is exposed. Tess' articulation and phonological development places her in Stage 3. Prominent error patterns in Tess' speech include Fronting, Stopping, Gliding, and Cluster Reduction.

SPEECH SAMPLE

See Appendix C–2.

QUESTIONS

1. Tess has difficulty pronouncing [k]. Develop a bombardment activity for [k] based on play with stuffed animals.

2. Develop a bombardment activity for [k] based on free play with assorted toys that contain [k].

3. Turn the above activity into a more structured one using a shoe box with a Cookie Monster face on the opening.

4. Suppose that Tess likes baseball. Develop a bombardment activity based on a bean bag tossing game.

5. Develop a bombardment activity for [k] based on a hide-and-seek game with pictures or cards.

6. For additional practice, develop a bombardment activity for [k] based on Tess and her favorite dolls going out to lunch.

7. Suppose you decide that each of the above activities requires too much time. Develop a quick bombardment activity for [k].

8. *For discussion:* Some clinicians recommend that the client wear a frequency modulated (FM) system during bombardment activities to increase the treatment target's saliency. What do you consider the merits and limitations of this recommendation?

Answer Sheet for Exercise 18–2: Bombardment

1. **Stuffed animals:**

2. **Assorted toys:**

3. **Cookie Monster:**

4. **Bean ball:**

5. **Hide-and-seek:**

6. **Lunch:**

7. **Quick activity:**

8. *For discussion:*

Exercise 18–3: Bombardment

This exercise focuses on developing bombardment activities for Billy, the client in Stage 4 whose speech was looked at in Section IV. Billy is 6 years, 11 months of age, is without cognitive impairments, and has a speech problem involving [r].

SPEECH SAMPLE

See Appendix C–8.

QUESTIONS

1. Billy has difficulty pronouncing [r]. Develop a bombardment activity for [r] based on tongue twisters.
2. Suppose Billy doesn't like tongue twisters (or the clinician finds them difficult to perform). Develop a bombardment activity for [r] based on poems or songs.
3. Develop a bombardment activity for [r] based on a game in which Billy is blindfolded.
4. For additional practice, develop a bombardment activity for [r] based on picture naming cards.
5. Develop a bombardment activity for [r] which includes reading Billy a story.

Answer Sheet for Exercise 18–3: Bombardment

1. **Tongue twisters:**

2. **Poems or songs:**

3. **Blindfold game:**

4. **Naming cards:**

5. **Story:**

CHAPTER
19

Increasing Awareness

Treatment generally proceeds more rapidly if a client is aware of the sounds and syllables that are the focus of remediation. The major techniques used to achieve this are metaphors, descriptions and demonstrations, and touch cues. The exercises in this chapter emphasize specialized activities to teach metaphors, and descriptions and demonstrations to less developmentally advanced clients. Touch cues, whose instruction requires more persistence of effort than specialized activities, are not discussed in the exercises.

METAPHORS

Metaphors compare some aspect of speech to something with which the client is familiar. For example, a metaphor for [s] is "the snake sound," and a metaphor for a fricative is "the long sound." Possible metaphors for sound classes, syllables, and characteristics of words are listed in Tables 19–1, 19–2, and 19–3 (Blodgett & Miller, 1989; Flowers, 1990).

DESCRIPTIONS AND DEMONSTRATIONS

Descriptions and demonstrations provide a simple means to heighten a client's awareness of selected characteristics of speech. A possible description of [p], for example, draws the client's attention to the closing lips, the buildup of air behind the lips, and the sudden release of air. A demonstration accompanying the description might involve placing a piece of paper in front of the client's lips to show the sudden release of air or gently pressing the client's lips together to show lip closure.

Touch Cues

Touch cues draw the client's attention to production characteristics of sounds (typically, the place of production). For example, a client might be instructed to touch the two lips for bilabial oral stops, to touch above the lips for alveolar stops, and to touch under the back of the chin for velar stops (Bleile & Hand, in press). Originally designed for clients with oral-motor dysfunction, touch cues are now finding their way into wider clinical use. Possible touch cues are listed in Table 19–4.

TABLE 19–1. Possible metaphors for different places of production.

Place of Production	Metaphors
Bilabial	Lip sounds
Labiodental	Biting lip sounds or biting sounds
Interdental	Tongue tip sounds
Alveolar	Bump sounds, hill sounds
Postalveolar	Back of the hill sounds
Palatal	Middle sound
Velar	Back sounds
Glottal	Throat sound

TABLE 19–2. Possible metaphors for different manners of production.

Manner of Production	Metaphors
Fricatives	Long sounds, hissing sounds
Glides and liquids (approximants)	Flowing sounds
Lateral	Side sound
Affricates	Engine chugging sounds
Nasals	Nose sounds
Stops	Short sounds, dripping sounds, and popping sounds
Voiced	Motor on, voice on, buzzing sound, hand buzzer sound, buzzing voice box, and voice box on
Voiceless	Motor off, voice off, not a buzzing sound, not a hand buzzer sound, no buzzing voice box, and voice box off

TABLE 19–3. Possible metaphors for consonant clusters, syllables, and words.

Sound Units	Metaphors
End of word	End sound
Multisyllabic words	Words with parts
Single syllable words	Words with one part
Initial consonants	Starting sounds
Consonant clusters	Sound friends

Compiled from "Easy Does It For Phonology" by E. Blodgett & V. Miller, 1989, East Moline, IL: LinguiSystems.

TABLE 19–4. Possible touch cues for different places and manners of production.

Sound class	Example	Touch cue
Nasals	[m]	• Fingers and thumb hold lips together; ask client to feel vibration on neck
	[n]	• Lay finger over front of cheek bone
Oral Stops	[p] [b]	• Lay finger in front of lips
	[t] [d]	• Lay finger above top lip
	[k] [g]	• Lay finger at upper most part of neck
Fricatives	[f] [v]	• Lay finger below bottom lip
	[θ] [ð]	• Place finger in front of lips and remind client to stick out tongue
	[s]	• Point to the corner of the mouth (to indicate spread) and remind client to close teeth gently
	[ʃ]	• Lay finger in front of lips and use the metaphor "quiet sound"
Liquid	[l]	• Place tip of finger at midline of top lip
Diphthongs	[oʊ]	• Trace finger around lips and use the metaphor "blowing sound"
	[eɪ]	• Place fingers on corners of mouth and use the metaphor "smiling sound"

Exercise 19–1: Increasing Awareness

Metaphors provide an important means to increase a client's awareness of speech. The present exercise offers the opportunity to develop a list of metaphors for individual sounds. The list can be derived from published sources, the clinician's own imagination, or a combination of both. Sources that contain relatively extensive lists of metaphors include Bleile (1995), Blodgett and Miller (1989), and Flowers (1990).

Selecting Metaphors

Whenever possible, involve the client in the selection of a metaphor. For example, if the treatment target is [s], ask the client what he or she wants to call that sound, offering possibilities such as the "snake sound," the "hissing sound," and the "whistling teakettle sound." Most clients in Stage 3 and almost all clients in Stage 4 are able to make such a decision.

QUESTIONS

1. For which stages in articulation and phonological development are the use of metaphors most appropriate?

2. Complete the table of metaphors by developing one or more metaphors for each of the consonants and [ɚ]. *The first sound is an example and is answered for you.*

Answer Sheet for Exercise 19–1: Increasing Awareness

1. **Stages:**

2. **Metaphors:**

Metaphors

Sound	Metaphors
[p]	Popping sound
[b]	
[t]	
[d]	
[k]	
[g]	
[f]	
[v]	
[θ]	
[ð]	
[s]	
[z]	
[ʃ]	
[ʒ]	
[tʃ]	
[dʒ]	
[m]	
[n]	
[ŋ]	
[l]	
[ɚ]	
[r]	
[j]	
[w]	
[h]	

Exercise 19–2: Increasing Awareness

Once the clinician and client select a metaphor, the clinician needs to make the metaphor "more real" for the client. To illustrate, if the client selects to call [s] the "snake sound," the clinician spends a few minutes explaining how the sound is like a snake because of its hiss, and so on. This exercise offers opportunities to practice brief descriptions of metaphors for individual sounds, sound classes, and syllable and word positions. The client whose speech forms the basis of this exercise is named Tess. Tess is 4 years, 4 months of age and is mildly delayed in both Korean and English, the two languages to which she is exposed. Prominent error patterns in Tess' speech include Fronting, Stopping, Gliding, and Cluster Reduction.

SPEECH SAMPLE

See Appendix C–2.

QUESTIONS

1. Tess has difficulty with velar sounds. Suppose [k] is a treatment target and develop a brief explanation for [k] as the "cawing crow sound." (**Hint:** As you answer this and the other questions in this exercise, remember that the metaphors are options. Few clinicians would simultaneously teach all the metaphors described below. *This is an example and is answered for you.*

2. Instead of the "cawing crow sound," suppose that Tess selects to call [k] the "coughing sound." Develop a brief explanation for that metaphor.

3. Fronting also affects Tess' pronunciation of postalveolar sounds. Suppose that Tess selects the "motor boat sound" as her metaphor for the voiced postalveolar fricative. Develop a brief explanation to explain this metaphor.

4. Suppose the clinician selects Stopping instead of Fronting. Suppose further that Tess selects to call [s] the "teakettle sound." Develop a brief description for this metaphor.

5. Many times a clinician wishes to have a metaphor for a class of sounds either in addition to or instead of a metaphor for an individual sound. Suppose that Tess selects "long sounds" as a metaphor for sounds such as [f], [v], [s], and [z] (fricatives). Develop an activity to explain the metaphor "long sound." (**Hint:** For this exercise, before teaching the metaphor, briefly describe how you will determine that Tess understands the concept of long.)

6. Sometimes a clinician needs a metaphor for a word or syllable position rather than for a sound or sound class. Tess has difficulty with word final consonants. Develop an activity to teach the metaphor "end sound" for consonants that end words.

7. Tess also has difficulty producing consonant clusters. Develop an activity to explain the metaphor of consonant clusters as "sound friends."

Answer Sheet for Exercise 19–2: Increasing Awareness

1. **Cawing crow sound:** Show Tess a picture of a large black crow and imitate the cawing sound it makes. Talk about crows and their significance to a farmer, explaining how scarecrows are supposed to keep crows away from the farmer's fields by making them think the farmer is out working in his field. Next, read a story about a crow, finding opportunities to make "cawing" noises during the reading.

2. **Coughing sound:**

3. **Motor boat sound:**

4. **Whistling teakettle sound:**

5. **Long sound:**

6. **End sound:**

7. **Sound friends:**

Exercise 19–3: Increasing Awareness

Brief descriptions and demonstrations of sounds are useful in increasing the speech awareness of selected clients in Stage 3 and most clients in Stage 4. The client whose speech sample serves as the basis for this exercise is Kelly, a child 5 years, 10 months of age whose speech contains Stopping of [s] and several other fricatives. The descriptions and demonstrations in this exercise all pertain to [s].

SPEECH SAMPLE

See Appendix 3–7.

QUESTIONS

1. Suppose that you and Kelly select the "whistling teakettle sound" as the metaphor for [s]. Develop a description of [s] incorporating that metaphor. The description should be understandable to a client near 6 years of age. (**Hint:** Your answer will be easier to write if you present your description verbatim.)

2. Simple demonstrations are often a useful adjunct when trying to increase a client's awareness of how a sound is produced. Develop a simple demonstration for the place of production of [s] using a lifesaver tied to a piece of dental floss. (**Hint:** Assume for this and the following questions that you wish to facilitate the variant of [s] that is produced with the tongue raised.)

3. If [s] is being facilitated with the tongue tip lowered, where is the lifesaver placed?

4. Instead of the above activity, develop a demonstration activity using chewing gum to facilitate Kelly's awareness of the alveolar place of production.

5. For additional practice, develop a simple demonstration for the place of production of [s] using the analogy of a ticking clock.

6. The above activities focus on the place of production of [s]. Develop a simple demonstration focusing on the manner of production of [s] using a tongue depressor or cotton swab and a mirror.

7. As a challenge, develop a simple demonstration focusing on the manner of production of [s] that relies only on verbal instructions.

8. Kelly often pronounces [s] as [t]. Develop a simple demonstration focusing on the manner of production of [s] based on Kelly's error pattern.

Answer Sheet for Exercise 19–3: Increasing Awareness

1. **Description of [s]:**

2. **Lifesaver:**

3. **Tongue lowered:**

4. **Chewing gum:**

5. **Ticking clock:**

6. **Tongue depressor and mirror:**

7. **Manner of production:**

8. **[t] to [s]:**

CHAPTER
20

Facilitating Syllables and Words

Activities designed to facilitate syllable and word development are used within many therapy approaches. Word pairs focus the client's attention on how speech errors influence communication. Facilitation of syllables and words offers a means to improve a client's syllable and word structure.

WORD PAIRS

Languages use sound to distinguish the meaning of words. The difference in meaning between *cup* and *pup*, for example, is that the former begins with [k] and the latter with [p]. Contrastive elements of sound facilitate perception and production through word pairs (also called minimal and maximal pairs), which are words that differ by a single sound (Tyler, Edwards, & Saxman, 1987; Elbert, Rockman, & Saltzman, 1982; Weiner, 1981). The words *bee-pea*, for example, are a word pair in which the words differ from each other by one sound, [b] and [p]. The

words *bee* and *pea* are a **minimal pair**, because they differ by a single distinctive feature (voicing) within most distinctive feature systems. Word pairs can also differ by more than one distinctive feature (called **maximal pairs**), as in *pea-me*, which differ in voicing ([p] is voiceless and [m] is voiced) and nasality ([p] is an oral consonant and [m] is a nasal consonant).

Some evidence suggests that use of maximal pairs is more effective with clients in the early stages of articulation and phonological development, and that minimal pairs may be more appropriate for clients in later stages of articulation and phonological development (Gierut, 1989). Word pairs may also differ in the presence or absence of a sound, such as in *bee-beet* and *slow-low*.

BUILDING SYLLABLES AND WORDS

Most facilitative techniques target sounds rather than syllables and words. Bernhardt (in press) has pioneered efforts to develop techniques to facilitate syllable and word development. Three specific techniques focus on final consonants, consonant clusters, and retention of syllables.

Final Consonants

Many clients have difficulty in using consonants to close syllables and words. A client, for example, might pronounce *beet* as [bi] through Final Consonant Deletion. Bernhardt recommends using a rhyming word task to remediate this error pattern (Bernhardt, in press). In such tasks, a client is first presented a story containing rhyming words ending in vowels. Once the client appears to grasp the concept of rhymes, rhyming words ending in consonants are introduced. The first story, for example, might involve *Pooh*, *Roo*, and cows that go *moo*, while the second story (or continuation of the first story) might involve a girl named *June* who sings a *tune* to the *moon* while standing on a *dune*.

Consonant Clusters

The acquisition of consonant clusters may present significant difficulty to certain clients. A client, for example, might pronounce *ski* as [ki] through Cluster Reduction. The remediation principle used to facilitate consonant cluster development is the same one that causes speakers to typically pronounce *is* as *tis* in phrases such as *it is* (Bleile, 1991). In such phrases, the final consonant ([t] in this case) tends to migrate to the following syllable if that syllable begins with a vowel. Similarly, a consonant cluster can be introduced into word-initial position through a phrase such as *ask a*, which, if said quickly enough, is likely to be pronounced as *a ska* (Bernhardt, in press).

Retention of Syllables

Even after a client is able to produce most sounds, he or she may still have difficulty retaining unstressed syllables in longer words, words with unusual stress patterns, and word compounds. A client, for example, might be able to say *in*, but may delete the same syllable when it occurs in a word such as *serendipity* through a developmentally advanced form of Syllable Deletion.

Remediation to retain syllables is accomplished in three steps (Bernhardt, in press). First, the client practices multisyllabic words, producing them with equal syllable intensities and durations. Next, the client is provided practice in alternating loud-soft and short-long syllables. Third, the client is taught to use key words and rhythm cues. The STRONG-weak-Strong stress pattern, for example, might be called *the elephant's beat*, and the weak-STRONG-weak stress pattern might be called *Aladdin's beat*. (Capital letters indicate primary stress.) A possible variation on this procedure is to use visual and tactile cues to illustrate the number of syllables in a word. A clinician, for example, might have the client place a bead on a string for every syllable in the word. A Hawaiian variation on this activity is to let the beads represent flowers on a lei (Imanaka-Inouye, 1994, personal communication).

Exercise 20–1: Facilitating Syllables and Words

Word pairs are the primary facilitative technique within many therapy approaches. This and the following exercise provides opportunities to develop word pair activities for perception and production. The client this exercise is based on is Tess, a child 4 years, 4 months of age whose speech was considered in Section IV. Tess is mildly delayed in both Korean and English, the two languages to which she is exposed. Prominent error patterns in Tess' speech include Fronting, Stopping, Gliding, and Cluster Reduction.

Activities for Perception and Production

Although some activities lend themselves better to either perception or production, the vast majority can be used for either purpose. To illustrate, a fishing game is a perceptual activity when the clinician names a picture for a client to "catch" with a hook, and a production activity when the clinician and client reverse roles. Similarly, barrier games and magic boxes are perceptual activities when the client is asked to identify the word said by the clinician and production activities when the client and clinician reverse roles.

SPEECH SAMPLE

See Appendix C–2.

QUESTIONS

1. What principle underlies the use of word pairs?

2. For which stage or stages in articulation and phonological development are word pairs appropriate?

3. Tess has difficulty with many fricatives. Develop a perceptual word pair activity for Tess based on a bean bag tossing game. Have the exercise focus on Stopping of [s]. (**Hint:** For this and the following questions focus more on describing the activity than on the specific words you will use in the game.) *This question is an example and is answered for you.*

4. For additional practice, develop a barrier game for the same treatment target as above.

5. Fishing games also provide good activities for word pairs. Develop a fishing game as a perceptual activity for Tess.

6. A "magic box" offers another way to develop a word pair activity. Develop a "magic box" as a perceptual activity for Tess.

7. Word pair activities can be used for production as well as perception. Develop a word pair activity to assist Tess with the production of [s], for which she uses a Stopping error pattern. Build the activity around a skit in which a puppet has difficulty saying words correctly and is always using a word that is "close" to the intended word but which definitely does not convey the intended meaning.

8. Tess also has difficulty with Gliding. Develop a production word pair activity based on a goat who only eats things whose names start with [r].

Answer Sheet for Exercise 20–1: Facilitating Syllables and Words

1. **Principle:**

2. **Stages:**

3. **Bean bag toss:** Place large picture cards representing word pairs such as *bus/bum* on the floor at least 18" apart. To verify that Tess knows the words, ask her to name the pictures. Ignore incorrect pronunciations and either select new pictures or teach the vocabulary for the pictures named incorrectly. Instruct Tess to throw a bean bag onto the picture you named. Alternately, tape picture pairs (such as *bus/bum*) on the wall, asking Tess to use the bean bag to hit each word you named.

4. **Barrier game:**

5. **Fishing game:**

6. **Magic box:**

7. **Puppets:**

8. **Goat:**

Exercise 20–2: Facilitating Syllables and Words

This exercise provides opportunities to develop word pair activities for a client in an early elementary grade. This exercise is based on Billy, the client in Stage 4 whose speech was considered in Section IV. Billy is 6 years, 11 months of age, no cognitive impairments, and has speech problems involving [r].

SPEECH SAMPLE

See Appendix C–8.

QUESTIONS

1. Develop a perceptual word pair activity for Billy. Base the activity on the clinician reading sentences aloud in which one word is missing. *This question is an example and is answered for you.*

2. Develop a Bingo game as the basis of a perceptual word pair activity for Billy.

3. For additional practice, develop a perceptual word pair activity for Billy based on listening to a story.

4. Develop a production activity using word pairs to remediate Billy's pronunciation of [r]. Base the activity on a turn-taking board game of your choice.

5. For additional practice, develop a table top billiard game into a production word pair activity.

6. A barrier game offers another option for a production word pair activity. Develop such an activity for Billy.

Answer Sheet for Exercise 20–2: Facilitating Syllables and Words

1. **Reading aloud:** Show Billy a picture while reading aloud a sentence that is missing one word. Provide Billy pictures of a word pair, asking him to point to the word that is left out. For example, the sentence might be, "The lookout point is dangerous. That's why they built a _____." The word pair is *rail* and *whale*. (**Note:** This activity can be adapted for an older client by not using a picture and having the client write his or her answer on an answer sheet.)

2. **Bingo:**

3. **Story:**

4. **Board game:**

5. **Billiards:**

6. **Barrier game:**

Exercise 20–3: Facilitating Syllables and Words

Many clients have significant difficulty mastering the structure of syllables and words. A number of activities focus directly on facilitating syllable and word development. The present exercise focuses on such activities for two clients, Tess and Billy, both of whom were discussed in exercises in Section IV.

SPEECH SAMPLES

See Appendices C–2 and C–4.

QUESTIONS

1. Tess often has difficulty pronouncing word final consonants. For example, *big, boat, down,* and *one* are all pronounced as syllables ending in vowels. Develop an activity using chalk and a chalkboard to facilitate Tess' ability to pronounce word final consonants.

2. Tess also has difficulty with beginning and ending syllables and words with consonant clusters. For example, *sticker* and *skate* are both pronounced without word initial consonant clusters. Develop an activity to facilitate Tess' acquisition of word initial consonant clusters beginning with [s]. Base the activity on a toy snake who hisses [s].

3. Tess occasionally has difficulty retaining syllables in words. For example, in *telephone* Tess pronounces the STRONG-weak-strong stress pattern as STRONG-weak. Develop a simple activity to facilitate Tess' perception of syllables. Base the activity on hand clapping or foot tapping.

4. Describe how you might convert the above activity into a production exercise.

5. List some activities other than clapping and tapping that you might use with Tess to indicate syllables in words.

6. While Billy does not have difficulty pronouncing [r] at the end of words, he does have difficulty pronouncing [r] in consonant clusters. Develop an activity to facilitate Billy's development of word initial consonant clusters containing [r]. Base the activity with turns selected by spinning a wheel.

7. The speech sample for Billy does not contain sufficient examples to know if he has difficulty pronouncing longer multisyllabic words. Suppose, however, that the results of a word probe indicates such a problem exists. Develop a connect-the-dots activity to facilitate this aspect of Billy's articulation and phonological development. Indicate briefly how the activity might be used to facilitate perception and then indicate briefly how it might be used to facilitate production.

8. List some additional activities you might use with Billy to help him recognize syllables in words.

Answer Sheet for Exercise 20–3: Facilitating Syllables and Words

1. **Chalkboard:**

2. **Snake:**

3. **Clapping or tapping:**

4. **Production:**

5. **Other syllable retention activities:**

6. **Spinning wheel game:**

7. **Connect-the-dots:**

8. **Other syllable retention activities:**

CHAPTER 21

Indirect and Direct Techniques

The exercises in this chapter focus on direct and indirect techniques used to facilitate articulation and phonological development. The body of indirect techniques is called facilitative talk and the two most widely used direct instruction techniques are phonetic placement and shaping.

FACILITATIVE TALK

Facilitative talk is a body of techniques for talking with clients who have articulation and phonological disorders and language disorders (Bleile, in press). For some clients facilitative talk is an adjunct to more direct instruction; for others it is the primary means of intervention. The principle options for facilitative talk include motherese, expansions, strategic errors, modeling, parallel talk, and requests for confirmation or clarification.

Motherese

Motherese is a combination of facilitative talk techniques that serve to capture and keep a client's attention. Motherese speech modifications include higher than usual pitch, talking about shared perceptions, exaggerated intonation, use of repetitions, and calling attention to objects.

Expansions

Expansions fill in incorrect or missing speech parts. The client, for example, might say [pi] for *bee*, and the clinician might repeat the word, changing [p] to [b]. Alternately, if the client deleted [t] in *beet*, the clinician might repeat after the client, expanding [bi] to [bit].

Strategic Errors

Strategic errors are clinician-produced speech errors that mimic aspects of the client's articulation and phonological disorder. If, for example, the client pronounces word-initial [t] as [d], during the course of play the clinician might point to a doll's toe and say, "Doe." The hoped-for response is that the client looks confused or laughs and then attempts to say the word with an initial [t].

Modeling

Modeling involves the use of the clinician, another person, or a favored toy as a speech example. In a modeling game, for example, the clinician might introduce a puppet as the teacher and have the client and clinician serve as the students. The puppet teacher instructs the students to repeat what the puppet says, which are words that contain the treatment target.

Parallel Talk

In parallel talk, the clinician talks about the client's actions and the objects to which he or she is attending. For example, with a client who has [b] as a treatment target, the clinician might fill the clinic room with objects whose names contain this sound. When the client looks at a ball, the clinician might say "ball," and as the client rolls the ball across the floor, the clinician might say, "Ball rolling" or "Here comes the ball."

Requests for Confirmation or Clarification

Requests for confirmation or clarification are techniques designed to focus a client's attention on the communicative adequacy of his or her speech. During play, for example, a client whose treatment target is [k] might say *key* as *tea*. The clinician might ask, "Did you say tea?" or "What did you say you wanted?" or "Did you say you wanted some tea?" or "I thought I heard you say tea. Is that what you meant

to say?" The hoped-for response is that the client will repeat, "Key" or say something like, "I said key."

PHONETIC PLACEMENT AND SHAPING TECHNIQUES

Phonetic placement and shaping techniques were the stock-and-trade of speech-language clinicians for much of the 20th century (Fairbanks, 1960; Nemoy & Davis, 1954). The use and knowledge of these techniques has declined in recent years, as client populations have shifted downward in age and increased in severity of involvement. Still, many clients benefit from careful use of phonetic placement and shaping techniques, especially the more cognitively advanced clients in Stage 3 and most clients in Stage 4.

Phonetic Placement

Phonetic placement techniques teach the tongue and lip positions used in speech production. Phonetic placement techniques to teach [t], for example, might include asking the client to raise the tongue tip, touch the tongue tip to the alveolar ridge, and to quickly draw the tongue tip down again.

Shaping

Shaping techniques use a sound the client can already produce (either a speech error or another sound) to learn a new sound. Shaping techniques, for example, provide a series of steps through which a client who says [w] is taught to say [r].

Exercise 21–1: Indirect and Direct Techniques

This and the following exercise provide opportunities to identify types of facilitative talk and to develop facilitative talk activities.

A Time-Honored Technique

Modeling is a time-honored facilitative technique that has been used by teachers in a wide range of disciplines. For example, it is used by golf instructors to teach a golf swing and by directors to teach actors to make dramatic entrances. The

principle is simple: "Watch and listen to what I do and to what I say and then copy me. I will give you feedback and then may ask you to perform the action again."

QUESTIONS

1. At which stage or stages in articulation and phonological development is facilitative talk most often used?

2. Why do you suppose that facilitative talk rather than direct instruction is used in those stages?

3. Which type of facilitative talk has the clinician providing examples for the client to repeat?

4. Which type of facilitative talk has the clinician pretending not to understand the client?

5. Which type of facilitative talk has the clinician talking about the actions and the objects to which the client is attending?

6. Which type of facilitative talk includes higher than usual pitch, talking about shared perceptions, exaggerated intonation, use of repetitions, and calling attention to objects?

7. Which type of facilitative talk involves the clinician filling in the missing parts in the client's speech?

8. Which type of facilitative talk involves the clinician imitating the client's incorrect productions?

9. *For discussion:* Describe in your own words the purpose of facilitative talk.

Answer Sheet for Exercise 21–1: Indirect and Direct Techniques

1. **Stages:**

2. **Facilitative talk:**

3. **Facilitative talk:**

4. **Facilitative talk:**

5. **Facilitative talk:**

6. **Facilitative talk:**

7. **Facilitative talk:**

8. **Facilitative talk:**

Exercise 21–2: Indirect and Direct Techniques

This exercise offers opportunities to develop facilitative talk activities. The speech on which this exercise is based is from a child named Matt (Carpenter, 1995). Matt is 2 years, 3 months of age and his development appears completely typical except in the area of articulation and phonology.

SPEECH SAMPLE

Intended Words	Matt
1. mama	mama
2. ball	ba
3. eyes	aɪ
4. bear	bɝ
	bɛr
5. bye bye	baɪbaɪ
	bʌbʌ
6. dog	dɑ
7. cake	geɪ
8. yeah	jæ
9. bus	bʌ
10. all	aʊ
11. kitty	gigi
12. mine	maɪ
13. Babette	bæbə
14. Kate	keɪkeɪkeɪ
15. moo	mun
16. wow	woʊ
17. apple	ʔæʔæ
18. duck	duʔ~
	dʌk
19. up	ʌ
20. yes	ɛs

9. *For discussion:*
QUESTIONS

1. Matt pronounces *bus* without a final consonant. Develop a short facilitative talk activity that uses expansion to promote Matt's pronunciation of a final consonant in *bus. This is an example and is answered for you.*

2. With clients of Matt's developmental level, requests for confirmation or clarification have the clinician pretending not to understand what the client says. Develop a simple activity involving requests for confirmation or clarification to promote Matt's pronunciation of *cake* (word 7).

3. Matt has difficulty pronouncing word final consonants. Develop a short parallel talk activity to help promote this aspect of speech.

4. Most often, facilitative talk techniques are employed in conjunction with each other rather than individually. Develop a telephone activity that incorporates motherese, expansion, and requests for confirmation or clarification. (**Hint:** For this exercise you need only show how you would incorporate these techniques into

the activity. You do not need to identify specific sounds and words you will use.)

5. Sometimes including another person in treatment helps the client understand that other people also make mistakes. Develop an activity with a puppet that incorporates at least strategic errors, expansion, and modeling.

6. For additional practice, design an arts and crafts activity that employs parallel talk and expansion.

Answer Sheet for Exercise 21-2: Indirect and Direct Techniques

1. **Bus activity:** Ask Matt if he wants to play. Bring out a toy garage, cars, and a bus. Place the bus toy next to you and ask Matt to tell you which toys he wants. When Matt says *bus* as "ba," say after him, "Bus" or something like, "Here's the bus."

2. **Cake activity:**

3. **Parallel talk activity:**

4. **Telephone activity:**

5. **Puppet activity:**

6. **Arts and crafts activity:**

Exercise 21–3: Indirect and Direct Techniques

This exercise provides you with the opportunity to develop phonetic placement and shaping techniques and activities. The exercise focuses on [s], a sound frequently facilitated through these techniques. The client is Kelly, the child whose speech was analyzed extensively in the previous section. Kelly's articulation and phonological development approximates that of a client in Stage 3. Kelly is 5 years, 10 months of age and her intellectual development is at least average.

Developing Phonetic Placement and Shaping Techniques

Two "tricks" are useful in developing phonetic placement and shaping techniques and activities. First, think about how a sound is produced. For example, [b] is produced with the lips closed and the vocal cords vibrating. Second, develop a metaphor or scenario that conveys in a simple way what you know about the sound's produc- tion. For example, the closed lips might be depict- ed as a closed castle drawbridge, and the vibrat- ing vocal cords might be depicted as a bee that is buzzing in your throat. Only the limits of a clini- cian's imagination define the number of possible ways to describe sounds.

SPEECH SAMPLE

See Appendix C–7.

QUESTIONS

1   For which clients are phonetic placement and shaping techniques most useful?

2. What is the difference between phonetic placement and shaping?

3. Develop a phonetic placement technique using snake puppets to teach Kelly the phonetic placement of [s]. *This question is an example and is answered for you.*

4. Suppose that Kelly does not like snakes and that she appears uneasy with the above activity. Develop an activity to teach the phonetic placement of [s] using a balloon. (**Hint:** Use the balloon as a metaphor for the client's mouth.)

5. For additional practice, develop a phonetic placement technique to teach [s] using the metaphor of the mouth as a teakettle.

6. For additional practice, develop a phonetic placement technique for [s] by having Kelly be a space scientist who must fire a missle (through her straw) to have it hit a target on another planet.

7. Suppose none of the above techniques proves successful. You are about to give up when Kelly comes into therapy full of excitement, telling you that her family rented the movie *Pocahontas* last night and that she wants to be an American Indian. Develop a phonetic placement technique for [s] using the theme of Poca- hontas being a scout for her tribe on a canoe journey down a river.

8. Kelly's speech contains Stopping of [s] and other fricatives. Instead of phonetic placement techniques, de- velop a shaping technique from [t] to teach [s] using a woodpecker metaphor for [t].

9. For additional practice, use the metaphor of a jackhammer that goes t-t-t-t to shape [s] from [t].

Answer Sheet for Exercise 21–3: Indirect and Direct Techniques

1. **Clients:**

2. **Phonetic placement and shaping:**

3. **Snake activity:** Show Kelly pictures of a snake to demonstrate how quickly a snake can move its tongue in and out of its mouth. Next, review the metaphor lesson for [s] as the "hissing" sound using a snake puppet (preferably one with a tongue) making hissing noises with its tongue out. Have a "mother" snake tell the other snake(s) that "it is not polite to stick out your tongue when you are talking to someone." Have the puppet snake continue to try hissing with the tongue inside while talking to Kelly. Next, have Kelly "hiss" with her tongue out and slowly pull the tongue back inside the mouth while continuing to "hiss" softly. The [s] sound should result.

4. **Balloon activity:**

5. **Teakettle activity:**

6. **Straw activity:**

7. **Pocahontas activity:**

8. **Woodpecker activity:**

9. **Jackhammer activity:**

References

Acevedo, M. (1991, November). *Spanish consonants among two groups of Head Start children.* Paper presented at the convention of the American Speech-Language-Hearing Association, Atlanta, GA.

Bernhardt, B. (in press). Phonological intervention techniques for syllable and word structure development. *Clinics in Communication Disorders.*

Bailey, S. (1982). *Normative data for Spanish articulatory skills of Mexican children between the ages of six and seven.* Unpublished master's thesis, San Diego State University, San Diego.

Bernhardt, B., & Gilbert, J. (1992). Applying linguistic theory to speech-language pathology: The case of non-linear phonology. *Clinical Linguistics and Phonetics, 6,* 123–145.

Bernthal, J., & Bankson, N. (1993). *Articulation and phonological disorders.* Englewood Cliffs, NJ: Prentice-Hall.

Bleile, K. (1987). *Regressions in the phonological development of two children.* Unpublished doctoral dissertation. University of Iowa, Iowa City.

Bleile, K. (1991). *Child phonology: A book of exercises for students.* San Diego: Singular Publishing Group.

Bleile, K. (1995). *Manual of articulation and phonological disorders.* San Diego: Singular Publishing Group.

Bleile, K. (in press). Language intervention with infants and toddlers. In L. McCormick, R. Schiefelbusch, & D. From-Loeb (Eds.), *Language intervention in inclusive settings: An introduction* (3rd Ed.). New York: Allyn & Bacon.

Bleile, K., & Hand, L. (1995). Metalinguistics. *Journal of Clinical Linguistics and Phonetics, 9,* 25–28.

Bleile, K., & Miller, S. (1994). Toddlers with medical needs. In J. Bernthal & N. Bankson (Eds.), *Articulatory and phonological disorders in special populations* (pp. 81–109). New York: Thieme.

Bleile K., Stark R., & Silverman McGowan, J. (1993). Speech development in a child after decannulation: Further evidence that babbling facilitates later speech. *Clinical Linguistics and Phonetics, 7,* 319–337.

Bleile, K., & Tomblin, J. (1991). Regressions in the phonological development of two children. *Journal of Psycholinguistic Research, 20,* 483–499.

Blodgett, E., & Miller, V. (1989). *Easy does it for phonology.* East Moline, IL: LinguiSystems.

Bodine, A. (1974). A phonological analysis of the speech of two Mongoloid (Down syndrome) boys. *Anthropological Linguistics, 16,* 1–24.

Braine, M. (1974). On what might constitute learnable phonology. *Language, 52,* 489–498.

Branigan, G. (1976). Syllabic structure and the acquisition of consonants: The great conspiracy in word formation. *Journal of Psycholinguistic Research, 5,* 117–133.

Carpenter, K. (1995). *Articulation and phonological exercises.* Unpublished masters' project, Division of Speech Pathology and Audiology, University of Hawaii, Honolulu.

Chomsky, N., & Halle, M. (1968). *The sound pattern of English.* New York: Harper and Row.

Cruttenden, A. (1978). Assimilation in child language and elsewhere. *Journal of Child Language, 5,* 373–378.

De la Fuente, M. (1985). *The order of acquisition of Spanish consonant phonemes by monolingual Spanish speaking children between the ages of 2.0 and 6.5.* Unpublished doctoral dissertation, Georgetown University, Washington, DC.

Diedrich, W. (1983). Stimulability and articulation disorders. In J. Locke (Ed.), *Seminars in Language Disorders, 4.*

Dunn, L., & Dunn, L. (1981). *Peabody picture vocabulary test—Revised.* Circle Pines, MN: American Guidance Service.

Dyson, A. (1988). Phonetic inventories of 2- and 3-year-old children. *Journal of Speech and Hearing Disorders, 53,* 89–93.

Elbert, M., & Gierut, J. (1986). *Handbook of clinical phonology: Approaches to assessment and treatment.* Austin, TX: PRO-ED.

Elbert, M., Powell, T., & Swartzlander, R. (1991). Toward a technology of generalization: How many exemplars are sufficient? *Journal of Speech and Hearing Research, 34,* 81–87.

Elbert, M., Rockman, B., & Saltzman, D. (1982). *The sourcebook: A phonemic guide to monosyllabic English words.* Austin, TX: Exceptional Resources.

Fairbanks, G. (1960). *Voice and articulation drill book.* New York: Harper & Row.

Fantini, A. (1985). *Language acquisition of a bilingual child: A sociolinguistic perspective* (to age 10). San Diego: College-Hill Press.

Ferguson, C., & Farwell, C. (1975). Words and sounds in early language acquisition: English initial consonants in the first fifty words. *Language, 51,* 419–439.

Ferguson, C., & Macken, M. (1983). The role of play in phonological development. In K. Nelson (Ed.), *Child language IV* (pp. 256–282). Hillsdale, NJ: Lawrence Erlbaum.

Ferguson, C., Peizer, D., & Weeks, T. (1973). Model-and-replica phonological grammar of a child's first words. *Lingua, 31,* 35–65.

Fey, M., & Gandour, J. (1982). Rule discovery in phonological acquisition. *Journal of Child Language, 9,* 71–82.

Flowers, A. (1990). *The big book of sounds.* Austin, TX: PRO-ED.

Gierut, J. (1989). Maximal opposition approach to phonological treatment. *Journal of Speech and Hearing Disorders, 54,* 9–19.

Goldman, R., & Fristoe, M. (1969). *Goldman-Fristoe test of articulation.* Circle Pines, MN: American Guidance Service.

Goldstein, B. (1988). *The evidence of phonological processes of 3- and 4-year-old Spanish-speakers.* Unpublished master's thesis, Temple University, Philadelphia.

Goldstein, B. (1995). Spanish phonological development. In H. Kayser (Ed.), *Bilingual speech-language pathology: An Hispanic focus* (pp. 17–38). San Diego: Singular Publishing Group.

Goldstein, B., & Iglesias, A. (in press). Phonological patterns in normally developing Spanish-speaking 3- and 4-year-olds of Puerto Rican descent. *Language, Speech, and Hearing Services in the Schools.*

Gonzalez, M. (1978). *Cómo detectar al niño con problemas del habla (Identifying speech disorders in children).* México: Editorial Trillas.

Gordon-Brannan, M. (1994). Assessing intelligibility: Children's expressive phonologies. *Topics in Language Disorders, 14,* 17–25.

Hodson, B. (1986). *Assessment of phonological processes—Revised.* Danville, IL: Interstate Publishers and Printers.

Hodson, B. (1989). Phonological remediation: A cycles approach. In N. Creaghead, P. Newman, & W. Secord (Eds.), *Assessment and remediation of articulatory and phonological disorders* (pp. 323–333). Columbus, OH: Charles E. Merrill.

Iglesias, A., & Anderson, N. (1993). Dialectal variations. In J. Bernthal & N. Bankson (Eds.), *Articulation and phonological disorders,* (3rd ed., pp. 147–161). New York: Prentice-Hall.

Ingram, D. (1975). Surface contrast in children's speech. *Journal of Child Language, 2,* 287–292.

Ingram, D. (1986). Explanation and phonological remediation. *Child Language Teaching and Therapy, 2,* 1–19.

Ingram, D. (1994). Articulation testing versus conversational speech sampling: A response to Morrison & Shriberg (1992). *Journal of Speech and Hearing Disorders, 37,* 935–936.

Ingram, D. (1989). *Phonological disability in children.* New York: American Elsevier.

International Clinical Phonetics and Linguistics Association. (1992a). The international phonetic alphabet. *Clinical Linguistics and Phonetics, 6,* 262.

International Clinical Phonetics and Linguistics Association. (1992b). Recommended phonetic symbols: Extensions to the IPA. *Clinical Linguistics and Phonetics, 6,* 259–261.

Izuka, K. (1995). *Articulation and phonological assessment with typically developing children aged 3:6 and 5:0.* Unpublished masters' project, Division of Speech Pathology and Audiology, University of Hawaii, Honolulu.

Kim, J. (1995). *Articulation and phonology exercises for students: Error patterns, dialect, and second language influence.* Unpublished masters' project, Division of Speech Pathology and Audiology, University of Hawaii, Honolulu.

Lee, K. (1994). *Case study analysis of articulation and phonological disorders in three children (stages 2–4).* Unpublished masters' project, Division of Speech Pathology and Audiology, University of Hawaii, Honolulu.

Ladefoged, P. (1983). *A course in phonetics.* New York: Harcourt, Brace, and Jovanovich.

Leinonen-Davies, E. (1988). Assessing the functional adequacy of children's phonological systems. *Clinical Linguistics and Phonetics, 2,* 257–270.

Leopold, W. (1947). *Speech sound development of a bilingual child: A linguist's record, vol. II: Sound-learning in the first two years.* Evanston, IL: Northwestern University.

Macy, A. (1979). *Normative data for Spanish articulatory skills of Mexican children between the ages of five and six.* Unpublished master's thesis, San Diego State University, San Diego.

Madison, C. (1979). Articulation stimulability review. *Language, Speech, and Hearing Services in Schools, 10,* 185–190.

Mason, M., Smith, M. & Hinshaw, M. (1976). *Medida española de articulación [Measurement of Spanish articulation].* San Ysidro, CA: San Ysidro School District.

McReynolds, L., & Kearns, K. (1983). *Single-subject experimental designs in communication disorders.* Baltimore: University Park Press.

Menn, L. (1976). *Pattern, control and contrast in beginning speech: A case study in the development of word form and word function.* Unpublished doctoral dissertation, University of Illinois, Champaign-Urbana.

Morrison, J., & Shriberg, L. (1992). Articulation testing versus conversational speech sampling. *Journal of Speech and Hearing Disorders, 35,* 259–273.

Morrison, J., & Shriberg, L. (1994). Response to Ingram letter. *Journal of Speech and Hearing Disorders, 37,* 936–937.

Nemoy, E., & Davis, S. (1954). *The correction of defective consonant sounds.* Magnolia, MS: Expression.

Peters, A. (1977). Language learning strategies: Does the whole equal the sum of the parts? *Language, 53,* 560–573.

Peters, A. (1983). *The units of language acquisition.* New York: Cambridge University Press.

Pollack, K. (1983). Individual preferences: Case study of a phonologically delayed child. *Topics in Language Disorders, 3,* 10–23.

Pollock, K., & Keiser, N. (1990). An examination of vowel errors in phonologically disordered children. *Clinical Linguistics and Phonetics, 4,* 161–178.

Powell, T. (1991). Planning for phonological generalization: An approach to treatment target selection. *American Journal of Speech-Language Pathology, 1,* 21–27.

Powell, T. Elbert, M., Dinnsen, D. (1991). Stimulability as a factor in generalization of misarticulating children. *Journal of Speech and Hearing Research, 34,* 1318–1328.

Robb, M., & Bleile, K. (1994). The phonetic inventory of children 1 to 2 years old. *Clinical Linguistics and Phonetics, 4,* 319–338.

Schwartz, R. (1988). Phonological factors in early lexical acquisition. In M. Smith & J. Locke (Eds.), *The emergent lexicon: The child's development of a linguistic vocabulary* (pp. 185–222). New York: Academic Press.

Schwartz, R., & Leonard, L. (1982). Do children pick and choose: An examination of phonological selection and avoidance in early lexical acquisition. *Journal of Child Language, 9,* 319–336.

Seo, R. (1995). *Exercises for articulation and phonological disorders: Assessment, analysis, and treatment.* Unpublished masters' project, Division of Speech Pathology and Audiology, University of Hawaii, Honolulu.

Shriberg, L. (1993). Four new speech and prosody-voice measures for genetics research and other studies in developmental phonological disorders. *Journal of Speech and Hearing Research, 36,* 105–140.

Shriberg, L., & Kwiatkowski, J. (1982). Phonological disorders III: A procedure for assessing severity of involvement. *Journal of Speech and Hearing Disorders, 47,* 256–270.

Shriberg, L., & Kwiatkowski, J. (1983). Computer-assisted natural process analysis (NPA): Recent issues and data. In J. Locke (Ed.), *Seminars in Speech and Language, 4,* 397.

Smit, A., Hand, L., Frelinger, J., Bernthal, J., & Byrd, A. (1990). The Iowa articulation norms project and its Nebraska replication. *Journal of Speech and Hearing Disorders, 55,* 779–798.

Smith, N. (1973). *The acquisition of phonology: A case study.* Cambridge: Cambridge University Press.

Stevens, K., & Keyser, S. (1989). Primary features and their enhancement in consonants. *Language, 65,* 81–106.

Stoel-Gamon, C. (1983). Constraints on consonant-vowel sequences in early words. *Journal of Child Language, 10,* 455–458.

Stoel-Gammon, C. (1985). Phonetic inventories, 15–24 months: A longitudinal study. *Journal of Speech and Hearing Research, 28,* 505–512.

Stoel-Gammon, C., & Dunn, C. (1985). *Normal and disordered phonology in children.* Baltimore: University Park Press.

Summers, J. (1982). *Normative data for Spanish articulation skills of Mexican children between the ages of four and five.* Unpublished master's thesis, San Diego State University, San Diego.

Task Force on Health Care. (1993). Task force on health care report. *Asha, 35,* 53–54.

Tyler, A., Edwards, A., & Saxman, J. (1987). Clinical application of two phonologically based treatment procedures. *Journal of Speech and Hearing Disorders, 52,* 393–409.

U.S. Bureau of the Census (1991). *Statistical abstract of the United States: 1991.* Washington, DC: U.S. Government Printing Office.

Van Riper, C. (1978). *Speech correction: Principles and methods* (6th ed.). Englewood Cliffs, NJ: Prentice-Hall.

Waterson, N. (1971). Child phonology: A prosodic view. *Journal of Linguistics, 7,* 179–221.

Weiner, F. (1981). Treatment of phonological disability using the method of meaningful minimal contrast: Two case studies. *Journal of Speech and Hearing Disorders, 46,* 97–103.

Williams, L. (1991). Generalization patterns associated with training least phonological knowledge. *Journal of Speech and Hearing Research, 34,* 722–733.

Wolfe, M. (1994). *Articulation and phonological exercises for students and clinicians.* Unpublished masters' project, Division of Speech Pathology and Audiology, University of Hawaii, Honolulu.

Yavas, M., & Lamprecht, R. (1988). Processes and intelligibility in disordered phonology. *Clinical Linguistics and Phonetics, 2,* 329–345.

APPENDIX
A

Answers to Exercises

Answers for Exercise 1–1: Distinctive Features

1. oral stops, fricatives, affricates
2. bilabials and labiodentals
3. [i ɪ eɪ ɛ æ a]
4. [s]
5. voice ([f] is voiceless and [v] is voiced)
6. voice and place ([p] is voiceless bilabial and [d] is voiced alveolar)
7. height ([i] is close and [eɪ] is close mid)
8. [ð]
9. [ʌ]
10. [j]
11. [r]
12. [p t k]
13. [i]
14. [w j l r]
15. [l]

Answers for Exercise 1–2: Distinctive Features

1. front, close mid, spread
2. lateral
3. voiceless oral stops
4. close, back, round
5. liquids
6. central
7. close, front, spread
8. close mid and open mid, front
9. approximants
10. front, between open mid and open
11. velar
12. voiceless sibilants
13. interdentals
14. alveolars
15. glides

Answers for Exercise 2–1: Speech Sounds

1. kæt
2. θɪn
3. junaɪt
4. bru
5. gɪvɪŋ
6. fɪŋgɚ neɪl pɑlɪʃ
7. sɛntʃɚi
8. pliz
9. wɪntɚ
10. bitwin

Answers for Exercise 2–2: Speech Sounds

1. dɔg
2. mʌni
3. sæt
4. dʒʌdʒ
5. mæstɚɪŋ
6. foʊnɛtɪk sɪmbʊlz
7. ʃip
8. laʊd
9. kɛtʃəp
10. jɛs

Answers for Exercise 3–1: Suprasegmentals

1. influence of an earlier sound on a later sound

2. influence of a later sound on an earlier sound

3. regressive assimilation; [n] (alveolar) assimilates toward the place of production of [θ] (interdental), causing [n] to be produced as a dental consonant

4. progressive assimilation; [r] (voiced) assimilates the voicing of [p] (voiceless), causing [r] to be produced as a voiceless consonant

5. regressive assimilation; [d] is deleted and [n] (alveolar) assimilates to the place of production of [w] (bilabial), causing [n] to be pronounced as [m] (bilabial)

6. progressive and regressive assimilation; [p] appears as a transition as the speaker's mouth moves from [m] to [θ] {[p] (bilabial) has the same place of production as [m] and the same voicelessness as [θ]}

7. progressive assimilation; [d] (alveolar) assimilates to the place of production of word-initial [b] (bilabial), causing [d] to be pronounced as [b] (bilabial)

8. regressive assimilation; [p] (bilabial) assimilates to the place of production of word-final [k] (velar), causing [p] to be pronounced as [k] (velar)

9. *For discussion:* regressive assimilation; [t] (alveolar) assimilates to the place of production of the following back vowel (back vowels are produced in the velar region), causing [t] to be pronounced as [k] (velar)

Answers for Exercise 3–2: Suprasegmentals

1. daɪ pɚ

4. bræn tʃɪz

2. pri tɛnd

5. æ bə loʊ ni

3. bə næ nə

6. wɪn tɚ

7. This is the syllable structure of *it is* when spoken slowly and carefully:

S S
Λ Λ
ɪt ɪz

When spoken quickly and casually, the syllable structure of the same phrase typically is:

S S
| Λ
ɪ tɪz

8. This is the syllable structure of *this time* when spoken slowly and carefully:

S   S
Λ Λ
ðɪs taɪm

When spoken quickly and casually, the syllable structure of the phrase often is:

S   S
Λ   Λ
ðɪ staɪm

9. *For discussion:* In both the above phrases, the final consonant of the first syllable moved to the beginning of the second syllable when the phrases were spoken quickly and casually. This mechanism can be used to facilitate the acquisition of word initial consonants and consonant clusters. For example, a "saying over" game can be used to facilitate word initial consonant clusters by having the client repeat the phrase *this time* over and over again in the hope that [s] in this moves to the beginning of *time*, creating a word initial [st] consonant cluster.

Answers for Exercise 3–3: Suprasegmentals

1. CV.CV
2. CVC.CV
3. VC.CV.CV.VC
4. V
5. CVC.CV

6. VC
7. VC
8. CV.CV.CVC. V.CV.CVCC
9. CCCVC
10. CVC

Answers for Exercise 3–4: Suprasegmentals

1. be GIN
2. BI shop
3. HA ppi ness
4. a STRO no my
5. TE le scope

6. MEA dow
7. FAIL ure
8. a PO lo gize
9. be LIE ver
10. astroPHYsics

Answers for Exercise 4–1: Modification to Symbols

1. [ls]
2. [m̥]
3. [ʔ]
4. [t˚]
5. [z̞]

6. voiced bilabial fricative
7. voiceless velar fricative
8. whistled
9. flap
10. velopharyngeal fricative

Answers for Exercise 4–2: Modification of Symbols

1. /k/
2. [k]
3. [p b]
4. [duk]
5. t → d
   d/t

6. liquids → glides
   glides/liquids
7. CC → CØ
   CØ/CC
8. g → k/___#
9. voiceless fricatives → voiced/V___V
10. The word two is pronounced tu~du.

Answers for Exercise 5–1: Phonetic Inventories

1. **Stress patterns:** Leslie's words are all stressed on the first syllable and the second syllable is unstressed. Judy's words are all single syllables (and, therefore, are stressed).

2. **Leslie:** Leslie's words are CV.CV.
   Judy: Judy's words are CV.

3. **Leslie:** All of Leslie's words have the following syllable structure: S
   /\
   CV

   Judy: All of Judy's words have the following syllable structure: S
   /\
   CV

4. **Leslie:** No consonants occur in two or more words.
   Judy: No consonants occur in two or more words.

5. **Leslie:** Leslie's phonetic inventory contains two vowels: a æ
   Judy: Judy's phonetic inventory contains one vowel: a

6. **Leslie:** Leslie's distinctive features for consonants are voiced (all consonants), bilabial ([m] and [b]), and oral stop ([b], [d], and [g]).
   Judy: Judy's distinctive feature for consonants is voiced (all consonants).

7. **Leslie:** Leslie's distinctive features for vowels are front (both vowels), open ([a]), and between open mid and open ([æ]).
   Judy: Judy's distinctive features for vowels are front and open ([a]).

8. **Similarities:** Leslie and Judy's phonetic inventories have similar syllable structures (CV), number of consonants in two or more words (none), the vowel [a], the distinctive feature of voicing for consonants, and the distinctive features of front and open for [a].
   Differences: Leslie and Judy's phonetic inventories differ in stress patterns of words (Leslie's words are stressed, unstressed and Judy's words are all stressed), sequence of syllables within words (Leslie's words are CV.CV and Judy's words are CV), vowel inventory (Leslie's inventory includes [æ]), distinctive features for consonants (Leslie's distinctive features include bilabial and oral stop) and distinctive features for vowels (Leslie's distinctive features include and between open mid and open for [æ]).

Answers for Exercise 5–2: Phonetic Inventories

1. **Davie:** n t p
   Child: none
2. **Davie:** VC, CV, CVC, CV.CV
   Child: CV, CV.CV
3.

Children	V	CV	CVC	VC
Davie:		✓	✓	✓
Child:		✓		

4. **Table 5–1:** b d h (3)
   Davie: b d k m ʃ (5)
   Child: b (l)

5.

Children	Stops	Nasals	Fricatives	Affricates	Glides	Liquids
Table 5–1:	✓				✓	
Davie:	✓	✓	✓			
Child:	✓					

6.

Children	Bi.	LabD.	InterD.	Al.	PostA.	Pal.	Vel.	Glot.
Table 5–1:	✓			✓				✓
Davie:	✓			✓	✓		✓	
Child:	✓							

7. Answer the following questions about common characteristics in development based on your answers to the previous questions.

   A. **Syllable structure:** CV
   B. **Consonant:** b
   C. **Manner of production:** stops
   D. **Place of production:** bilabial

8. A. Types of consonants: Norms = b d h
                            Davie = b d k m ʃ
                            Child = b

   B. Number of consonants: Norms = 3
                             Davie = 5
                             Child = 1

   C. Manners of production: Norms = stops, glides
                              Davie = stops, nasals, fricatives
                              Child = stops

   D. Places of production: Norms = bilabial, alveolar, glottal
                             Davie = bilabial, alveolar, postalveolar, velar
                             Child = bilabial

Answers for Exercise 5–3: Phonetic Inventories

1. **Hildegard:** p t b d g m n h j w
2. **Table 5–1:** t k b d g m n f s h w
   Hildegard: p t b d g m n h j w
   Kylie: p t b d m n f s z h j w
   Amahl: p b d g m n w l
   Jake: p t k b d g m n f s ʃ dʒ h j w
3. **Table 5–1:** 11
   Hildegard: 10
   Kylie: 12
   Amahl: 8
   Jake: 15

4.

Children	Stops	Nasals	Fricatives	Affricates	Glides	Liquids
Table 5–1:	✓	✓	✓	—	✓	—
Hildegard:	✓	✓	—	—	✓	—

continued

4. *continued*

Children	Stops	Nasals	Fricatives	Affricates	Glides	Liquids
Kylie:	✓	✓	✓	—	✓	—
Amahl:	✓	✓	—	—	✓	✓
Jake:	✓	✓	✓	✓	✓	—

5.

Children	Bi.	LabD.	InterD.	Al.	PostA.	Pal.	Vel.	Glot.
Table 5–1:	✓	✓	—	✓	—	—	✓	✓
Hildegard:	✓	—	—	✓	—	✓	✓	✓
Kylie:	✓	✓	—	✓	—	✓	—	✓
Amahl:	✓	—	—	✓	—	✓	✓	—
Jake:	✓	✓	—	✓	✓	✓	✓	✓

6. A. **Typical consonant inventory:** t k b d g m n f s h w
   Child with typical inventory: none

   B. **Average:** 11
   Range: 9 to 15

   C. **Typical:** stops, nasals, fricatives, and glides
   Range: Hildegard has the fewest number of different manners of production in her consonant inventory (stops, nasals, glides). Jake has the greatest number of different manners of production in his consonant inventory (stops, nasals, fricatives, an affricate, and glides.)

   D. **Typical:** bilabial, a labiodental, alveolar, velar, and a glottal.
   Range: Amahl has the smallest number of different places of production in his consonant inventory (bilabial, alveolar, a palatal, and a velar). Jake has the greatest number of different places of production in his consonant inventory (bilabial, a labiodental, alveolar, postalveolar, a palatal, velar, and a glottal.)

7. **For discussion:** An analysis of correctly pronounced sounds is not very informative for children in Stage 2, because such children pronounce most sounds incorrectly. When such an analysis is performed, the typical result is a short list (perhaps even none) of correctly pronounced sounds and a long list of sounds that the child cannot expected to pronounce correctly for many years.

Answers for Exercise 5–4

1.

Consonants	15 Months	24 Months
Norms:	b d h	t k b d g m n f s h w
Children:	b d k m ʃ	p t b d g m n f s h j w

2.

Number of Consonants	15 Months	24 Months
Norms:	3	11
Children:	1 to 5	9 to 15

3.

Manners	15 Months	24 Months
Norms:	stops & glides	stops, glides, nasals, & fricatives
Children:	stops, nasals, & fricatives	stops, glides, nasals, & fricatives

4.

Places	15 Months	24 Months
Norms:	bilabial, alveolar, & glottal	bilabial, labiodental, alveolar, velar, & glottal
Children:	bilabial, alveolar, postalveolar, & velar	bilabial, labiodental, alveolar, palatal, velar, & glottal

Answers to Exercise 6–1: Error Patterns

1. **Slash:** A slash above a vowel indicates that the syllable with the vowel carries primary stress.
2. **Multisyllabic:** words 6, 7, 14, 15, 17
3. **Primary stress:** Stress falls on the second syllable, except for *daddy* and *apple*, for which primary stress falls once on the first syllable and once on the second syllable.
4. **Error pattern:** Primary stress is moved from the first to the second syllable.
5. *Happy* and *bubble:* Primary stress will occur on the second syllable.
6. *For discussion:* Although there is no "right" answer to this question, here are two of many possibilities. First, Davie likely heard many words with stress on the second syllable (the word *banana*, for example). At some unconscious level, perhaps Davie hypothesized, based on words like *banana*, that all multisyllabic words should be pronounced with primary stress on the second syllable. Secondly, perhaps Davie began producing primary stress on the second syllable as sound play, and this became his regular way of saying multisyllabic words.

Answers for Exercise 6–2: Error Patterns

1. **Error pattern:** Final Consonant Deletion
2. **Exception:** *cake*
3. **Possible words:** *bait* and *mope*
4. **Words:**
   1. eɪ → i
   4. eɪ → i
   5. eɪ → i
   8. eɪ → i
   9. eɪ → i
5. **Affected vowel:** [eɪ] is pronounced as [i]
6. **Distinctive features:** close mid front → front close +spread
7. *hay* and *duke:* If the hypothesis is correct, *hay* should be pronounced [hi] and the vowel in *duke* should be unaffected.

Answers for Exercise 6–3: Error Patterns

1. **Error pattern:** Velar Assimilation
2. **Error pattern:** Labial Assimilation
3. **Place of production:** alveolar
4. **Assimilation:** Labial Assimilation
5. **Hypothesis:** When a word contains a velar and alveolar consonant, the alveolar consonant undergoes Velar Assimilation. When a word contains a labial and alveolar consonant, the alveolar consonant undergoes Labial Assimilation. When a word contains a velar and labial consonant, the velar consonant undergoes Labial Assimilation.
6. A. g g
   B. b b
   C. p p
   D. p b

7. **Hypothesis:** The first consonant in the word is added to words beginning with vowels.
8. **Possible words:** *eagle* (first sound = g) and *only* (first sound = n)

Answers for Exercise 6–4: Error Patterns

1. **Syllable initial consonants:** 5
2. **Place of production change:** Bilabial consonants are pronounced as alveolar consonants (words 4, 6, 7, 8, 10).
3. **Vowels:** [ɪ] and [i]
4. **Hypothesis:** Bilabial consonants are pronounced as alveolar consonants when followed by a front close vowel.
5. **Meet, bit, and bat:** The first consonants in *meet* and *bit* will be pronounced as [d] and [n], respectively, and the first consonant in *bat* will be pronounced as [b].
6. **Alternative hypothesis:** The error pattern probably does not involve all close vowels, because [u] in word 5 (*boo*) is a close vowel and in that word [b] is not pronounced as [d].

Answers to Exercise 6–5: Error Patterns

1. **Diacritic:** the consonant is syllabic
2. **Sound class:** nasal consonants
3. **Hypothesis:** The nasal consonant agrees in place of production of the preceding consonant.
4. **Mud and bib:** The final consonants will be [n] and [m], respectively.
5. **Hypothesis:** Nasal consonants are added to words ending in voiced oral stops, but not words ending in voiceless oral stops.
6. **Words ending in [k]:** A consonant will not be added.

Answers for Exercise 6–6: Error Patterns

1. **Manner of production:** Liquids
2. **Error pattern:** Gliding
3. **Exception:** *lamby*
4. **Error pattern:** Gliding (same name)
5. **Error pattern:** Stopping
6. **Notation:** liquids → glides/#___

Answers to Exercise 6–7: Error Patterns

1. **Error pattern:** Prevocalic Voicing
2. **Exceptions:** *poor, pretty, toothbrush, two, train*
3. **Word numbers:** 21–26, 29, 30
4. **Words:** *cake, cracker*
5. **Word:** *cookies*
6. **Error pattern:** Nasalization
7. **Notation:** unvoiced oral stops → voiced/#___

Answers for Exercise 6–8: Error Patterns

1. **Error patterns:** Cluster Reduction and Gliding
2.

driving

Ages	Word Initial Position	Intervocalic Position
1. 2;3	Cluster Reduction Gliding	Stopping
2. 2;5	Cluster Reduction	—
3. 2;7	—	—

3. **Word initial error patterns:** Prevocalic Voicing and Stopping
4. **Word final error patterns:** Stopping and a voiceless consonant is voiced at the end of words (for convenience, henceforth this simply is called Voicing)
5.

sauce

Ages	Word Initial Position	Word Final Position
1. 2;4	Prevocalic voicing Stopping	Voicing Stopping
2. 2;5	Prevocalic voicing Stopping	Stopping
3. 2;8	Stopping	Stopping
4. 2;11	(1) Stopping (2) Affrication (3) —	Stopping Affrication Affrication
5. 3;0	—	—

Answers to Exercise 6–9: Error Patterns

1. **Error pattern:** Gliding
2. **Error pattern:** Epenthesis
3. **Phonetic environment:** consonant clusters
4. **Words:** *grass, strawberry, string*
5. **[kr] consonant clusters:** *creep, crack, cross*
6. **Phonetic environment:** in isolation
7. **Consonant clusters:** [gl] (*glass*) and [sl] (*sled*)
8. **[fl] consonant cluster:** *flew, float, flower*

Answers for Exercise 6–10: Error Patterns

1. **Words:** 2, 4, 6, 7, 12
2. **Intended words:** 2, 4, 6, 7, 12
3. **Error pattern:** Word initial unstressed syllables either are deleted or sounds within the syllable are deleted when the following syllable receives primary stress.
4. **Stress pattern:** trochaic stress pattern
   Yes. Ryan's speech errors all occurred in words in which the primary stress occurs in the second syllable.
5. **Error pattern:** Syllable Deletion

Answers for Exercise 7–1: Consonants and Consonant Clusters

1. **Consonant classes:** stops, nasals, glides
2. **Fricatives:** [f]
3. **Consonant classes:** affricates, liquids, and all fricatives except [f] and those produced interdentally
4. **Consonant classes:** interdental fricatives
5. **Consonant clusters:** consonant clusters that begin with a voiceless stop and end in [w]
6. **Consonant clusters:**
   (1) consonant clusters with two members that begin with [s]
   (2) consonant clusters with two members whose second member is a liquid (exception: [θr])
   (3) a consonant cluster with three members whose third member is a glide
7. **Consonant clusters:**
   (1) [θr] and [tr]
   (2) consonant clusters with 3 members whose third member is a liquid
8. **Words:** *me, chew* and *glue* (same age), *spray*

Answers for Exercise 7–2: Consonants and Consonant Clusters

1.
Word Initial Consonants at 2 Years of Age

Sound	Smit et al.	Hildegard	Kylie	Amahl	Jake
p	✓		✓		✓
t	✓		✓		✓
k	✓				✓
b	✓	✓	✓	✓	✓
d	✓	✓	✓		✓
g	✓			✓	✓
m	✓	✓*	✓	✓	✓
n	✓	✓	✓	✓	✓
f	✓		✓		✓
θ					
s					✓
ʃ					
v					
ð					
z		✓			
tʃ					✓
dʒ					
h	✓		✓		✓
j	✓		✓		✓
w	✓	✓	✓	✓	✓
l					
r					

* = The pronunciation of Milwaukee is thought to result from deletion of the initial syllable.

2. A. **Smit et al.:** 12
   Hildegard: 6
   Kylie: 10
   Amahl: 5
   Jake: 14

   B. **Smit et al.:** all six oral stops, both nasal stops, and all three glides
   Amahl: one bilabial and one velar voiced oral stop, both the nasal stops, and one glide ([w])
   Jake: all six oral stops, both nasal stops, all three glides, and both alveolar fricatives

C. **Fricatives:** Smit et al's information indicates that children typically acquire [f] as their first consonant before 3 years of age. Of the four children, two (Hildegard and Amahl) have not yet acquired any fricatives, one child (Kylie) has acquired [f] as her only fricative, and one child (Jake) has acquired three fricatives ([f], [s], and [z]).

3. **Consonants:** [j] and [r]
4. **Sound class:** approximants
5. **Word:** *rope*
6. **Description of error:** [r] is pronounced with a [w]-like quality, which probably means lip rounding occurred
7. **Error pattern:** Gliding
8. **Consonants:** [s] and [r]
9. [s̺] = lisping of [s]
   [r̹] = w-coloring (lip rounding) of [r]

Answers for Exercise 7–3: Consonants and Consonant Clusters

1. **Kylie** = [sp st sn]
   Jake = [sp st sm sn sw]
2. No. Children vary in this as in other domains in articulation and phonological development.
3. **Word Initial [fl], [kl], and [kr] Consonant Clusters**

Clusters	Smit et al.	Rikki	Diane	Taylor	Tony
kl			✓		✓
kr			✓		✓
fl	✓		✓	✓	✓

4. [fr] is typically acquired by 3 years, 6 months. Of the four children, three have acquired [fr]. [kl] and [kr] are typically acquired by 4 years, 0 months. However, two of the four children aged 3 years, 6 months already have acquired these consonant clusters.
5. **Word Initial [spl], [spr], and [skr] Consonant Clusters**

Clusters	Smit et al.	Ryan	Shannon	Max	Puuala
spl	✓	✓	✓		✓
spr	✓	✓	✓		✓
skr	✓	NT*	✓		✓

* = not tested

6. All three consonant clusters are typically acquired by 5 years, 0 months of age. Of the four children, three have acquired all the consonant clusters and one child has acquired none of them. Information on one consonant cluster for one child (Ryan [skr]) is missing.

Answers for Exercise 8–1: Dialect

Intended Words	Child	AAEV Pattern(s)
1. bathe	bev	Place change
2. pen	pɪn	Raising of [ɛ] before nasals
3. house	haʊs	none
4. spoon	spū	Vowel nasalization

(continued)

(continued)

Intended Words	Child	AAEV Pattern(s)
		Deletion
5. skates	sket	Deletion
6. stars	sta.əz	Deletion
7. zipper	zɪpo	Deletion
8. keys	kiz	none
9. that	dæt	Stopping
10. shoe	ʃu	none
11. egg	ɛk	Devoicing
12. station	steʃæ̃	Vowel nasalization
		Deletion
13. fish	fɪʃ	none
14. sandwich	sæmwɪtʃ	none
15. thumb	θʌm	none

Answers for Exercise 8–2: Dialect

1. **Words:** *thumb, thorn, those, the mouse*
2. **Stopping:** Stopping as a dialect pattern is part of the language of a child's community, and Stopping as an error pattern indicates a difference between the speech of a child and his or her community.
3. **HC pattern:** *thread, throw, strap, string*
4. **Words:** *drum*
5. **Hypothesis:** [r] is typically produced with the tongue retracted, which "pulls" the preceding consonant further back in the mouth.
6. *For discussion:* It is important to avoid treating dialect as a disorder. Because Stopping of interdental fricatives is part of the community's language system, you should consider Stopping of interdental fricatives as a dialect pattern and should consider Stopping of other consonants as an error pattern.
7. *For discussion:* This is a controversial topic. I share the concern of many who worry that treatment for dialect reduction confirms the suspicion of some persons that dialect is a type of disorder. Nonetheless, I provide this service because, in my opinion, the client's right to clinical care outweighs other considerations.

Answers for Exercise 8–3: Dialect

Intended Words	Child	SIE Pattern(s)
1. van	bæn	Stopping
2. beads	bits	Consonant Devoicing
3. cheese	tʃis	Consonant Devoicing
4. green	griŋ	Nasal Velarization
5. yellow	dʒelo	Affrication
6. feather	fedor	Stopping
7. fish	fitʃ	Affrication
8. glove	glʌb	Stopping

(continued)

(continued)

Intended Words	Child	SIE Pattern(s)
9. ice cubes	aɪkjups	Consonant Devoicing
10. jump rope	tʃʌmrop	Consonant Devoicing
11. mouth	mat	Stopping
12. Jason	dʒesoŋ	Nasal Velarization
13. Santa Claus	santaklas	Consonant Devoicing
14. shoe	tʃu	Affrication
15. spoon	spũŋ	Nasal Velarization

Answers for Exercise 8–4: Dialect

Intended Words	Child	SIE	Developmental
1. pillow	pɪwo		l → w
2. toothache	tutek	Stopping	
3. feather	fɛdo	Stopping	
4. hello	xeho		l → x
5. football	tʊtbal		f → t
6. zebra	sibra	Devoicing	
7. cowboy	taʊbɔɪ		k → t
8. office	apɪs		f → p
9. movie	mubi	Stopping	
10. book	bʊt		k → t

Answers for Exercise 8–5: Dialect

Intended Words	Child	Likely	Unlikely	Dialect	English
1. boka	oka		✓		mouth
2. xaβon	haβon			✓	soap
3. floɾ	foɾ	✓			flower
4. dos	dot		✓		two
5. deðo	eðo		✓		finger
6. maɾtijo	mattijo			✓	hammer
7. gato	gago		✓		cat
8. xuɣo	kuɣo	✓			juice
9. kasa	kata		✓		house
10. bloke	boke	✓			block
11. weβo	welo		✓		egg
12. tɾen	tɾem		✓		train

Answers to Exercise 9–1: Acquisition Strategies

1. **Strategy:** word-based learning
2. **Strategy:** gestalt learning
3. **Strategy:** regression
4. **Strategy:** homonym seeking
5. **Strategy:** homonym avoiding
6. **Strategy:** word recipes
7. **Strategy:** selectivity

Answers for Exercise 9–2: Acquisition Strategies

1. **Stress patterns:** All the words contain a stressed syllable followed by an unstressed syllable.
2. **Sequence of syllables:** All the words are CV.CV.
3. **Place of production:** bilabial, alveolar, velar
4. **Manner of production:** oral and nasal stops
5. **Vowels:** [i] (word final position)

Answers for Exercise 9–3: Acquisition Strategies

1. **Distinctive features:** The consonant is voiced, palatal, and nasal.
2. **First recipe:** 1, 2, 4, 6, 9
   Second recipe: 3, 5, 7, 8
3. **Stress pattern:** Yes. All the words are monosyllables. Therefore, the words are all stressed, as the child does not yet put words in sentences.
4. **Syllables:** No. Some words begin with consonants; others do not.
5. **Consonants and vowels:** The common consonant is the word final postalveolar voiceless fricative. There are no common vowels.
6. **Distinctive features:** The common distinctive features for consonants are those of the word final consonant (postalveolar, fricative, voiceless). The common distinctive feature for vowels is vowel height between close and close mid.
7. **Word recipe:** Words within this recipe are single syllables that end in [ʃ] and have vowels whose height is between close and mid close.
8. A. **Stress:** The first syllable is stressed, the second is unstressed.
   B. **Sequence of syllables:** CV.CV
   C. **Consonants:** [ɲ]
   D. **Vowels:** front
   E. **Consonant distinctive features:** palatal, nasal, voiced
   F. **Vowel distinctive features:** none
9. **Word recipe:** Words within this recipe are two syllables in length, contain front vowels, and have the palatal nasal as their only consonant.

Answers for Exercise 9–4: Acquisition Strategies

1. **Primary stress:** the second syllable
2. **Date:** on 1;7.24
3. **Description:** Jacob begins pronouncing *kaka* with primary stress on the first syllable.

4. **Primary stress:** the first syllable
5. **Dates:** The regression begins on 1;7:10 and ends on 1;8:10.
6. **Regression:** Jacob begins pronouncing *cracker* and *cookie* with primary stress on the second syllable.
7. *Cackle*: with primary stress on the second syllable
8. **Explanation:** If Jacob's problem is a physical problem in producing primary stress on the first syllable, he should pronounce *kaka* with primary stress on the second syllable.
9. *For Discussion:* There is, of course, no one right answer to this question. Note that Jacob's regression is similar to Davie's error pattern affecting stress (Exercise 2–5). Perhaps for Jacob—as may have been the case for Davie—the change in stress represents a type of sound play.

An alternate explanation similar in spirit to that offered by Menn (1976) is that Jacob's regression may have arisen as an attempt by the child's articulation and phonological system to find a common way to pronounce stress patterns in three similarly sounding words. To illustrate, prior to 1;6:27, Jacob's articulation and phonological systems may have had one means of stress in *kaka* (place primary stress on the second syllable) and another way for stress *cracker* and *cookie* (place primary stress on the second syllable). Jacob's regression represents an attempt to pronounce stress for all three words in a similar way (primary stress on the second syllable). For several weeks Jacob pronounces all three words with stress on the second syllable, which results in the regression of *cracker* and *cookie*. However, a result of this new systematic way for pronouncing primary stress is that Jacob's pronunciation of *kaka*, *cracker*, and *cookie* sound less like the models in his community, leading him to revise his way for saying stress on the first syllable for *cracker* and *cookie*. The regression of *kaka* is not yet undone by 1;8:22, which is the end of the study.

If the above possible explanation seems far-fetched, recall that similar overgeneralization of rules lead to regressions in morphological development in children near 4 years of age. For example, a 4-year-old child who for months may have said *gave*, *bought*, and *slept* may develop a rule to regularize such irregular past tense verbs into *gived*, *buyed*, and *sleeped*.

Answers for Exercise 10–1: Measures of Severity and Intelligibility

1. **Severity score:** approximately 2.7 (round to 3, which indicates moderate degree of severity)
2. **Severity score:** approximately 2.3
3. A.

Word Numbers	Attempted	Correct
1.	2	2
2.	1	1
3.	2	1
4.	2	2
5.	2	1
6.	2	1
7.	2	2
8.	1	1
9.	2	2
10.	1	1
11.	3	0
12.	1	1
13.	2	1
14.	3	1
15.	2	1
16.	2	1
17.	4	4
Total:	**34**	**23**

3. B. **PCC:** approximately 67% (a mild to moderate disorder)
4. approximately 46%
5. *For discussion:* Clinical judgment scales have the merits of being easy and quick to administer, two important characteristics in settings in which speech-language clinicians evaluate and treat large numbers of clients. A major weakness of clinical judgment scales is that they are highly subjective, leading to situations in which the same client might be el-

igible for treatment in one setting but not in another. The PCC is the best researched method for determining severity. A limitation of the PCC is that its reliance on spontaneous speech makes its use difficult in most clinical settings.

Percentage of development offers a speedy means to calculate severity of involvement. A limitation of percentage of development is that it ignores individual differences in development. It also is probably more accurate to say that a client's speech is similar in some respects to a younger person's speech than saying that the client's speech is a certain percentage below his or her chronological age.

6. *For discussion:* The answers to this question are probably as varied as the clinicians who treat articulation and phonological disorders. I think all agree on the need for a method to establish eligibility for treatment, and that, at least for the time being, severity fulfills that important purpose. A difficulty with measures of severity is that the criteria to determine treatment eligibility often seems arbitrary. For example, which level of severity, number of factors involved, or percentage of development must be met before a person is determined to be eligible to receive articulation and phonological care? Is mild severity sufficient? Or must the severity be moderate or severe? Must one factor be present? Or more than one? Must a person be 25% delayed? Or 10%? Or 50%? The difficulty in answering these questions in a nonarbitrary way is that little research exists on how severity relates to future articulation and phonological development.

A related issue to consider is that persons with the same severity rating may have different prognoses for future articulation and phonological development. To illustrate, the speech of three potential clients might be judged to be mildly disordered, but only one may have a medical history that suggests he or she is at high risk for speech problems in the future. In this situation, even though the scores of all three children are similar, most clinicians more willingly provide treatment to the individual with a poorer prognosis for future articulation and phonological development.

Answers for Exercise 10–2: Measures of Severity and Intelligibility

1. A. **Intelligibility score:** approximately 1.3 (round to 1, which indicates readily intelligible)
   B. **Intelligibility score:** approximately 3.7 (round to 4, which indicates mostly intelligible)
2. A. **Treatment target:** [s] because it ranks fourth in relative frequency, with [z] ranking fifteenth
   B. **Treatment target:** [s] because it ranks highest in relative frequency compared to other voiceless fricatives
   C. **Treatment target:** [k] because it ranks higher in relative frequency than [l]
3. A. **Error pattern:** Fronting, because it has greater effect on intelligibility
   B. **Error pattern:** [k] because it ranks higher in relative frequency than [g]
   C. **Error pattern:** Final Consonant Deletion gives the listener less information about the word being attempted than does Fronting. To illustrate, when Final Consonant Deletion occurs in a word such as *beak*, the listener has no evidence that the word he or she is trying to understand ends in a consonant. However, when Fronting occurs in a word such as *beak*, the listener knows the word ends in a consonant, even though he or she may not know which consonant is being attempted.
4. *For discussion:* Their merits and limitations are similar to those for clinical judgment scales of severity. Both types of clinical judgment scales are speedy and easy to use, but are also highly subjective.
5. *For discussion:* Both methods have the important advantage of attempting to address the effects of treatment on intelligibility. A limitation of all the methods is that a person's intelligibility reflects not only the relative frequency of sounds or error patterns, but also reflects such variables as the setting in which speech occurs, the speaker's appearance, and the listener's familiarity with the speaker's topic. Additionally, few clinicians use intelligibility as the sole criterion in treatment target selection. Other aspects of speech that are typically considered include developmental age norms and the client's better abilities.

Answers to Exercise 11–1: Developmental Age Norms

1. **Word initial consonants:** [b g]
2. **Word final consonants:** none
3. **Common distinctive features:** Both consonants are voiced oral stops.
4. **Different distinctive features:** place of production. [b] is bilabial and [g] is velar.
5. **Age equivalence:** 15 months
6. **Words:** probably *bug*, as the word initial consonant and the vowel are already in Johnny's phonetic inventory

Answers for Exercise 11–2: Developmental Age Norms

1. **Word initial:** b d g m
2. **Word final:** none
3. **Age equivalence:** In terms of number and type of consonants, Matt's consonant inventory resembles that of a child near 15 months of age. Matt's consonant inventory contains four consonants in word initial position and none in word final position. The speech of a child near 15 months of age is expected to contain approximately three consonants in word initial position and none in word final position. Additionally, in common with children near 15 months of age, the majority of the consonants in Matt's inventory are voiced oral stops.
4. **Matt's Consonant Inventory**

| | Inventory | |
Criterion	Word Initial	Word Final
1 word	k b d g m j w	n ʔ k s
2 word	b d g m	none
3 word	b m	none

5. *For discussion:* The answer to this question depends on the clinician's purpose. If a clinician wishes to identify all the consonants a client produces, a criterion of one word might be most appropriate. A criterion of two words seems more appropriate when the clinician wishes to identify those consonants that occur more widely in the client's speech. Similarly, a criterion of three words (or, for that matter, four, five, or six words) is useful when the clinician only wishes to identify consonants that occur widely in a client's speech. Of course, the result of increasing the number of words in which a consonant must occur is that the clinician will identify ever fewer consonants as being acquired. Although none of the above criteria are inherently better or worse than the others, most clinicians select two or three words as their criteria to avoid either use of rarely occurring consonants (which can happen if a criterion of one word is used) or excluding consonants that occur fairly widely in a small expressive vocabulary (which can occur if a criterion of four or more words is used).

Answers for Exercise 11–3: Developmental Age Norms

1. **Word initial:** t d g h ḅ
2. **Word final:** m
3. **Age equivalence:** 12 months of age

Answers for Exercise 11–4: Developmental Age Norms

1. **Error pattern:** Fronting
   Example: cannot
2. Tess is 4 years, 4 months of age and her speech contains error patterns that typically occur in the speech of children less than 3 years of age.
3. If developmental age norms are the sole treatment criterion, Fronting should be the treatment focus, because it is not expected to occur in the speech of children beyond 3 years of age, although Stopping is expected to continue in children over that age.
4. **Possible words:** *cap, bug, key, go, pick*
5. **Category:** present

Answers for Exercise 11–5: Developmental Age Norms

1. **Error pattern:** Stopping
2. yes
3. **Calculation of Percentage of Occurrence**

Words	Dora	Stopping
4. telephone	bæbən	1/1
5. tricycle	taɪtɪtoʊ	1/1
14. bananas	næenəz	0/1
18. bus	bʌs̩	0/1
21. blocks	bwɑʃ	0/1
23. give	dɪb	1/1
26. monster	mɑnsə	0/1
30. fishing	pɪʃɪn	1/2
31. feathers	pɛɾəs	2/3
32. fits	bɪts	1/2
33. find	faɪn	0/1
34. scissors	tɪzɔz	1/3
35. sun	tʌn	1/1
36. soap	soʊp	0/1
37. socks	ʃɑʃ	0/2
38. stop	tɑp	0/1
39. sleeping	pipɪn	1/1
40. shovel	s̩ʌbl̩	1/2
44. zoo	su	0/1
45. zipper	ti	1/1
56. leaf	wif	0/1
61. ice cream	aɪtim	0/1
Total:		12/30
Percentage: 40%		

4. **Category:** present
5. **Word Probe**

Words	Dora	Stopping
1. sun	tʌn	1/1
2. fun	pʌn	1/1
3. bus	bʌs	0/1
4. zoo	s̩u	0/1
5. maze	meɪz	0/1
Total:		2/5
Percentage: 40%		

6. **Category:** present
7. *For discussion:* The merit of the longer word list is that the results are based on a larger speech sample, and its limitation is that the larger sample size requires a longer amount of time to analyze. The word probe approach has the opposite merits and limitations: It is quick to use, but is based on a smaller speech sample. In the present example, the two procedures yield similar results. A worthwhile study for future research would be to determine the extent to which the two procedures provide comparable results across a number of clients in various stages in articulation and phonological development.

Answers for Exercise 11–6: Developmental Age Norms

1. **[r]:** 50% = 3;6
   75% = 6;0

2. Billy is 6 years, 8 months old. Approximately 50% of children are expected to produce [r] correctly by 3 years, 6 months of age, and approximately 75% are expected to pronounce [r] correctly by 6 years, 0 months.

3. **Developmental Age Norms for Consonant Clusters**

Consonant Clusters	Developmental Age Norms	
	50%	**75%**
kr	4;0	5;6
br	3;6	6;0
dr	4;0	6;0
gr	4;6	6;0

4. Billy is 6 years, 8 months old. Approximately 75% of children are expected to produce [r] correctly by 6 years, 0 months of age in three of the four consonant clusters that were tested; the other consonant cluster is expected to be produced correctly by 75% of children by 5 years, 6 months.

5. **Word Probe**

Words	Billy	Correct
1. rain	reɪn	1/1
2. row	woʊ	0/1
3. run	ɾʌn	0/1
4. root	rut	1/1
12. row	woʊ	0/1
15. ring	ɾɪŋ	0/1
17. ray	ɾeɪ	0/1
Total:		2/7
Percentage:		28%

6. **Category:** emerging

Answers for Exercise 11–7: Developmental Age Norms

1. **Correct:** p t b d m n f s ʃ v z tʃ dʒ h l w
   Incorrect: k g j r

2. **Correct:** p t b d g m n ʃ z s v
   Incorrect: k f tʃ dʒ

3. **Correct:** none
   Incorrect: kr kl br fl st sn sl

4. Dee is 7 years, 5 months of age and produces several consonants in error that are typically produced correctly by children under 3 years of age. For example, Dee produces the following sounds incorrectly: word initial [k] and [g] and word final [k] and [f]. Dee also produces a number of sounds in error that are expected to be produced correctly by preschoolers between 3 and 5 years of age. Examples of these sounds include [r], [j] in *yellow*, and the word initial consonant clusters [kr kl br fl st sn sl].

5. **Word probe:** *you, yes, young* (a possible alternative is to include a word containing [l] —such as *yelling*— to determine if [j] typically is pronounced as [l] when both sounds occur in the same word)

6. **Word probe:** *spill, space, spy*

Answers for Exercise 12–1: Better Abilities

1. **Error Pattern:** Fronting
2. **Stimulability results:** Stacy was stimulable for the voiceless postalveolar friactive.
3. **Words:** *show, bush, cheap, beach, Jeep, edge*
4. **Phonetic placement technique:** A simple phonetic placement technique involves touching the client's tongue with a tongue depressor just behind the tip and then asking the client to raise that part of the tongue toward the roof of the mouth while puckering the lips and breathing out.
5. **Shaping:** A simple technique is to ask the client to say [s]. While the client is saying [s], ask him or her to pucker the lips slightly and to draw the tongue back a little until [ʃ] results.
6. *For discussion:* The primary merit of stimulability testing is that it provides a quick, simple method to assess if a client has some capacity to imitate a potential treatment target. Although stimulability is effective with most clients, not all clients are able to perform stimulability tasks, with others having no sounds in their speech for which they are stimulable, and still others have significant difficulty learning to produce stimulable treatment targets in spontaneous speech. A concern raised by some researchers is that client who is stimulable for a treatment target might make progress even without any treatment. Research on this important concern is equivocal (Diedrich, 1983; Madison, 1979; Powell, Elbert, & Dinnsen, 1991).
7. *For discussion:* Brief trials of phonetic placement and shaping techniques are valuable in determining if a client is likely to benefit from these methods during treatment. Because successful use of phonetic placement and shaping techniques requires the client to have relatively advanced cognitive and attention abilities, use of these techniques is generally limited to selected clients in late Stage 3 and in Stage 4. Another limitation of phonetic placement and shaping techniques is that clients typically require a number of steps to go from producing a sound using these techniques to producing a sound in spontaneous speech.

Answers for Exercise 12–2: Better Abilities

1. **Error pattern:** Prevocalic Voicing
2. **Exception:** *Pop Pop*
3. Yes. E produces [p] and [k] in word final position.
4. A. **Possible key word:** *Pop Pop*
   B. **Possible key environment:** word final position
5. A. **Yes/no:** Yes
   B. **Yes/no:** No

Answers for Exercise 12–3: Better Abilities

1. **Error pattern:** Fronting
2. **First bet:** Yes, syllable and word final positions
3. Yes
4. **Words:** *key, girl*
5. **Key word results:** Bobby will pronounce the first consonant in *key* and *girl* more accurately than in the other words.
6. **Chance results:** Bobby will pronounce the first consonant in *key* and *girl* no more accurately than in other words.
7. **Words:** Yes, in *Quick, clock, green, grow,* and *glue*
8. No
9. *For discussion:* A possible phonetic explanation is that Johnny pronounces all the cluster words with [w], a sound produced with the back of the tongue raised in the velar region. If this answer is correct, the key phonetic environment is a word initial velar consonant followed immediately by [w].

10. *For discussion:* A primary merit of these analyses is that they provide yet another means to identify potential treatment targets for which a client demonstrates some capacity to pronounce. As with other analyses of better abilities, when key environments and key words exist in a client's speech, they are more "first bets" than guarantees of treatment success. Lastly, although experienced clinicians are able to perform most key environment and key word analyses in a few minutes, those with less experience sometimes find these analyses both time consuming and challenging.

Answers for Exercise 13–1: Related Analyses

1. **Adjusted age:** 1 year, 3 months
2. **Adjusted age:** The client's adjusted age is the same as her chronological age (2 years, 3 months of age).
3. **Rationale:** Adjusted age is a better measure of developmental potential than is chronological age for children born prematurely. To illustrate, a full-term child is born following 9 months of in utero development, with a child born 2 months prematurely having 2 months less to develop. Adjusted age determines that a child's development is by the amount of time since conception, rather than the amount of time since birth.
4. Research indicates that children born prematurely have largely "caught up" in neurological development (to the extent they can catch up) to their chronological peers by 24 months of age.
5. $$\frac{57 \times 47}{100} = 26.79 \text{ months} = 2 \text{ years, 2 months of age}$$
6. In the latter situation, the client probably would not be considered to have an articulation and phonological disorder, because his articulation and phonological development is appropriate for his developmental age.
7. Most clinicians would say that the client does not have an articulation and phonological disorder, because his speech is appropriate to his level of development as represented by his language reception abilities.
8. *For discussion:* In persons without intellectual impairments, a person's potential for articulation and phonological development is established by his or her chronological age. For example, a child who is 4 years of age is expected to have the articulation and phonological abilities of a child near that age. Developmental age determination is useful for clients with intellectual or cognitive impairments, because chronological age typically does not well represent the articulation and phonological potential of such persons. To illustrate, a 9-year-old child with Down syndrome whose intelligence quotient is 43 is not expected to have the same articulation and phonological development as another child of his chronological age. The concept of developmental age attempts to best describe the articulation and phonological potential for such persons.

   An important question to consider is whether developmental age is an accurate representation of a person's articulation and phonological potential. Stated differently, if a person's language reception abilities approximates that of a child near 2 years of age, does that mean the person's potential for articulation and phonological development is that of a 2-year-old? Some persons with autism, for example, appear to have articulation and phonological abilities in advance of their other cognitive abilities. Relatedly, a common experience of many clinicians is that the articulation and phonological abilities of some persons with mental retardation always falls behind other cognitive domains, regardless of the amount of therapy, suggesting developmental age does not represent such persons' real potential.

Answers for Exercise 13–2: Related Analyses

1. **Sentences:**

   (1) **AAEV Pattern(s):** Place Change (n/ŋ in *playing*)
   Place Change (f/θ in *with*)
   Vowel Nasalization & Deletion (in *wagon*)
   Errors: d/dʒ (*Jerry*)
   d/dr (*drum*)
   φ/b (*ball*)
   d/g (*wagon*)

(2) **AAEV Pattern(s):** Place Change (n/ŋ in *making*)
   Errors: ø/h (*he*)
       ø/z (*is*)
       t/k (*making*)
       ʃ/tʃ (*much*)
       ø/z (*noise*)

(3) **AAEV Pattern(s):** Stopping (d/ð in *mother*)
                   Vowel Nasalization & Deletion (in *him*)
   Errors: t/k, ø/s (*makes*)
       t/st (*stop*)

(4) **AAEV Pattern(s):** Vowel Nasalization & Deletion (in *time*)
                   Place change (f/θ in *bath*)
   Errors: ʔ/t (*it*)
       ʔ/s (*is*)
       Ø/t (*it*)
       Ø/z (*is*)
       d/t (*take*)
       t/k (*take*)
       v/b (*bath*)

(5) **AAEV Pattern(s):** Stopping (d/ð in *the*)
   Errors: Ø/z (*lose*)
       t/p (*soap*)

2. *For discussion:* An important value of a picture description task is that it provides information about how a client talks in sentences. The primary limitation of such tasks is that sentences often require longer to analyze than single words.

Answers for Exercise 13–3: Related Analyses

Intended Words	Child	SIE	Errors
1. pencils	kɛnsɪls	Consonant Devoicing	p → k
2. matches	nates	Consonant Devoicing	m → n
			tʃ → t
3. drum	drʌt	—	m → t
4. duck	dʌt	—	k → t
5. shovel	tʃʌbəl	Affrication	—
		Stopping	
6. rabbit	rabit	—	—
7. carrot	kæwɪt	—	r → w
8. pajama	pitʃama	Consonant Devoicing	—
9. orange	orintʃ	Consonant Devoicing	—
10. stove	sob	Stopping	st → t
11. feather	felo	—	ð → l
12. blue	bu	—	bl → b

Answers for Exercise 13–4: Related Analyses

1. **Bilabial** **Alveolar** **Glottal**
      13   2   1

2. **Bilabial** = 81%
3. **Expected relative frequency** = 17.8%
4. **Strategy:** E's speech shows selectivity. E generally selects to attempt words that begin with bilabial consonants.
5. *For discussion:* See the discussion of selectivity in Chapter 6.

Answers for Exercise 13–5: Related Analyses

1. **(no answer)**
2. **Strategy:** word recipes
3. **Word numbers:** 1, 2, 4, 5, 7, 8, 10
4. **Word numbers:** 3, 6, 9
5. **Stress:** As both word recipes contain only monosyllables, the words in both recipes are stressed.
   Sequence of syllables: The words in both recipes consist of a single CV syllable.
   Consonant distinctive features: The consonants in words in both recipes are alveolar and voiced.
6. **Consonants:** The recipes differ in consonants. Words in the first recipe begin with [d], and words in the second recipe begin with [n].
   Consonant distinctive features: The consonant in the first word recipe is oral and the consonant in the second word recipe is nasal.

Answers for Exercise 14–1: Goals

1. **Long-term goal:** The long-term goal is for the client's articulation and phonological development to be appropriate to her chronological age.
2. **Long-term goal:** The long-term goal is for the client's articulation and phonological development to be appropriate to his developmental age.
3. **Long-term goal:** The long-term goal is for the client's articulation and phonological development to be appropriate to his adjusted age.
4. **Long-term goal:** The long-term goal is for the client's articulation and phonological development to be appropriate to her chronological age. Adjusted age is not calculated for children over 24 months of age. This problem highlights the rather arbitrary nature of the cutoff for adjusted age being 24 months.
5. **Long-term goal:** The long-term goal is for the client's articulation and phonological development to be appropriate to his chronological age.
6. **Long-term goal:** The long-term goal is for the client's articulation and phonological development to be appropriate to her developmental age. (In this case, developmental age rather than months of prematurity appears to best establish the client's expected "ceiling" for articulation and phonological development.)
7. **Long-term goal:** The long-term goal is for the client's articulation and phonological development to be appropriate to his adjusted and developmental age. (The goal might be written using either adjusted or developmental age, as they are equivalent in this situation.)
8. **Long-term goal:** The long-term goal is to eliminate the error pattern ([w] for [r]) causing the client to be teased.

Answers for Exercise 14–2: Goals

1. **Short-term goal:** reduction in interword variability
2. **Short-term goal:** maximize established speech abilities
3. **Short-term goal:** eliminate errors causing homonyms
4. **Short-term goal:** error pattern approach
5. **Short-term goal:** reduction in intraword variability
6. **Short-term goal:** flooding
7. **Short-term goal:** distinctive feature approach

Answers for Exercise 14–3: Goals

1. A. **Error pattern:** Prevocalic Voicing (1–4)
                           Cluster Reduction (2)
    B. **Error pattern:** Final Consonant Deletion (1, 2, 4)
    C. **Error pattern:** spreading of [ɪ]
2. A. **Error patterns:** Prevocalic Voicing (5, 6, 7, 11)
                            Fronting (6, 7, 8, 9, 11)
                            Stopping (8, 9, 10, 11)
    B. **Error patterns:** Syllable Deletion (6, 7, 9, 11)
                           Final Consonant Deletion (5, 8, 10)
    C. **Error pattern:** [ɔɑæ] – [a]
3. *For discussion:* There is no "correct" way to select which error pattern should be a short-term goal, although some error patterns are "better bets." To illustrate, although vowels are generally acquired earlier than most consonants, the vowel error patterns are not likely early candidates for short-term goals, because vowels have less impact on intelligibility than consonants and, further, little is known at present about how best to treat vowel errors.

    Syllable Deletion is a less than optimal short-term goal because it involves a wide number of diverse sounds and syllable structures, which limits the possibility that generalization will occur. Of the remaining error patterns (Stopping, Final Consonant Deletion, Fronting, and Prevocalic Voicing), Prevocalic Voicing may be the "best bet" for a short-term goal, both because it affects a number of words and because it typically is suppressed early in development. However, any of the other three error patterns are also reasonable choices and any might be selected as a short-term goal after considering such factors as stimulability, effect on intelligibility, the presence of key words, or social factors such being important to a client or his or her family.
4. **[bi]:** *beep, bee*
    [da]: *cat, dog*
5. *For discussion:* A first step in both short-term goals is to identify errors that result in homonyms. Either short-term goal can be undertaken using error patterns or sound classes based on distinctive features. The first short-term goal seeks to reduce homonyms by eliminating the error patterns or sound class errors that result in homonyms. Flooding works by causing communication frustration, which puts additional pressure on the client to reorganize how he or she speaks to be better understood.

Answers for Exercise 14–4: Goals

1. **Long-term goal:** Gavin's articulation and phonological development will be appropriate for his level of cognitive development.
2. **Options for short-term goals:** reduce homonyms, reduce variability, maximize established speech abilities, and eliminate errors affecting sound classes.
3. **Reduce homonyms:** Yes. Gavin's speech contains a number of homonyms. Two particularly common homonyms are [bʌ] and [dʌ]. The error pattern giving rise to the homonyms is described in answer to a question that follows.
4. **Reduce variability:** Yes, especially intraword variability. The following words contain a variant that is produced correctly: *pig, cat, door, fish, fan, cheese, house, rabbit.*
5. **Maximize established speech abilities:** Yes, if Gavin appears stalled in articulation and phonological development, or if the clinician wishes to focus on expanding Gavin's expressive vocabulary concurrent with articulation and phonological treatment.
6. **Elimination of errors affecting sound classes:** Yes. Error patterns in word initial position in three or more words include Fronting, Stopping, and Cluster Reduction. Fronting and Cluster Reduction occur 100% of the time and Stopping occur 90% of the time (the exception was the first sound in *sandwich*. The error pattern affecting vowels is Vowel Neutralization. One word (*sandwich*) is an exception out of 35 words, with Vowel Neutralization therefore occurring approximately 97% of the time. The error pattern in word final position is Final Consonant Deletion. It occurs 100% of the time.
7. *For discussion:* There are, of course, many "right" answers to this question. In considering the above options, I am struck that the error patterns occur largely without exception, suggesting that Gavin might find that short-term goal difficult. For the same reason, elimination of error patterns causing homonyms might also prove difficult for Gavin. This leaves three options: flooding, reduce variability, and maximization of established speech abilities. Although all

the three options are plausible short-term goals, flooding depends on causing Gavin communicative frustration, which might prove discouraging to Gavin, especially in the early phases of treatment. Maximization, too, might prove frustrating, because Gavin's phonetic inventory is so limited in syllable structures, consonants, and vowels that words developed through maximization are likely to be homonyms with existing words.

For all the above reasons, I would select to reduce variability as a first short-term goal, the rationale being that Gavin is more likely to have some early treatment success with this short-term goal, as he displays some capacity to pronounce the sounds on which treatment will focus. Successful reduction in variability would stabilize [æ], [f], [h], and the voiceless affricate. I would expect the next short-term goal to include elimination of errors affecting sound classes, especially Stopping, which should have several exceptions with reduction in variability. However, if the reduction in variability goal could not be met, I would consider flooding as a short-term goal.

Answers for Exercise 14–5: Goals

1. **Long-term goal:** Kelly's articulation and phonological development will be appropriate for her chronological age.
2. **Reduce homonyms:** No. Kelly's speech sample contains only a few homonyms. For example, *star* and *saw* are homonyms.
3. **Reduce variability:** No. Kelly's speech sample shows neither extensive intraword or interword variability. For example, the only words pronounced variably are *nose* and *rain*.
4. **Maximize established speech abilities:** No. Kelly does not appear stalled in articulation and phonological development, and her expressive vocabulary appears appropriate to her chronological age.
5. **Elimination of errors affecting sound classes:** Yes. Kelly's speech is notable for several error patterns, including Stopping, Gliding of liquids and [f], and Cluster Reduction. Affrication of fricatives occasionally affects words ending in [s] and [ʃ].
6. **Stopping (7/10)** = frequent
   Gliding (6/10) = frequent
   Cluster Reduction (8/10) = highly frequent
   Affrication (2/5) = present
7. *For discussion:* I would likely accept all four error patterns for short-term goals. Stopping affects a large class of sounds. Further, elimination of Stopping might reduce the occurrence of Cluster Reduction in consonant clusters containing fricatives. Gliding affects several sounds, including [f], which is typically acquired early in development. Cluster Reduction seems likely to prove challenging for Kelly, as it occurred so frequently. Lastly, although Affrication was of relatively low occurrence and affected only a few sounds in word final position, it might be included as a short-term goal to provide Kelly a balance of challenging and more easily mastered short-term goals.

Answers for Exercise 14–6: Goals

1. **First possible long-term goal:** Billy's articulation and phonological development will be appropriate for his chronological age.
   Second possible long-term goal: Treatment will eliminate articulation and phonological errors causing Billy to be teased.
2. **Short-term goal:** elimination of errors affecting late- acquired consonants, consonant clusters, and unstressed syllables in more difficult multisyllabic words
3. **Late-acquired consonants:** Yes. Billy produces [r] with [w] coloring in a number of words, including *ring, rabbit, drum,* and *American flag.*
4. **Consonant clusters:** Yes. Billy sometimes experiences difficulty with consonant clusters containing [r]. For example, *green* and *cry* are pronounced with word initial [gw] and [kw], respectively, and *great* is pronounced with word initial [gr].
5. **Unstressed syllables:** Although Billy does not appear to have difficulties with unstressed syllables in words included in the speech sample, the sample of longer multisyllable words is relatively small. For example, tested words include *pajamas, telephone,* and *American flag,* but does not include more scientific words such as *astronomy* and *umbilical.* If the clinician is concerned about this short-term goal, he or she could develop short word probes containing multisyllabic words.
6. **Word initial (nonclusters):** emerging
   Word initial (in clusters): rare

7. *For discussion:* The most likely short-term goal is word initial [r] both in and outside of consonant clusters. Most clinicians would likely establish word initial [r] outside of consonant clusters as a first short-term goal, on completion followed by word initial [r] in consonant clusters. A question raised by the analysis is if more information is needed about Billy's pronunciation of unstressed syllables in longer multisyllabic words. However, a satisfactory answer is difficult to reach until we have normative information on when children without speech problems are expected to pronounce such words correctly.

Answers for Exercise 15–1: Treatment Targets

1. **Long-term goals and treatment targets:** Treatment targets are the sounds and syllables for which the client receives treatment. Long-term goals are the behaviors that the client is expected to obtain at the end of treatment or a certain designated period of time, such as a semester or school year.
2. **Short-term goals and treatment targets:** Treatment targets are the sounds and syllables for which treatment is provided. Short-term goals are the steps, typically lasting from 2 to 4 weeks, through which long-term goals are obtained.
3. **Long-term goal:** The long-term goal is for the client's articulation and phonological development to be appropriate to his or her adjusted age.
   Short-term goals: The short-term goal is to reduce homonomy through flooding.
   Treatment target: [bi]
4. **Long-term goal:** The long-term goal is for the client's articulation and phonological development to be appropriate to his or her developmental age.
   Short-term goals: The short-term goals are to reduce Fronting and Stopping.
   Treatment targets: The treatment targets are [k] and [f].
5. **Long-term goal:** The long-term goal is for the client's speech to be appropriate to his or her chronological age.
   Short-term goal: The short-term goal is to eliminate Gliding of [r].
   Treatment target: The treatment target is [r].

Answers for Exercise 15–2: Treatment Targets

1. **Technique:** flexibility
2. **Technique:** most knowledge method
3. **Technique:** emerging sound
4. **Technique:** training deep
5. **Technique:** time (cycles)
6. **Technique:** key word
7. **Technique:** least knowledge method
8. **Technique:** stimulability
9. **Technique:** training wide
10. **Technique:** percentage
11. **Technique:** phonetic placement and shaping

Answers for Exercise 15–3: Treatment Targets

1. **Most knowledge method:** The treatment target is word initial [p], because this sound only differs minimally from [b]. Both [b] and [p] are bilabial oral stops, but [b] is voiced and [p] is voiceless.
2. **Least knowledge method:** The treatment target is [k], because this sound differs in several features from sounds already in E's phonetic inventory. All of E's word initial consonants are voiced bilabial or alveolar stops. In the process of facilitating [k], E also acquires two distinctive features: velar and unvoiced.
3. **Most knowledge method:** The treatment target is [t], as its features are most similar to those already in E's phonetic inventory. Both [d] and [t] are alveolar oral stops, but [d] is voiced and [t] is voiceless.

4. **Least knowledge method:** The treatment target is [s], because in acquiring [s] E also acquires the fricative and unvoiced features.
5. **Most knowledge method:** The treatment target is [s], as (compared to [f]) its distinctive features are most similar to those already in E's expressive vocabulary. Both [d] and [s] share a common place of production (alveolar), but differ in voicing and manner of production.
6. **Least knowledge method:** The treatment target is [f], because in acquiring [f] E also acquires a new place of production (labiodental), a new manner of production (fricative), and a voicing contrast ([f] is voiceless and the other word initial consonants in E's phonetic inventory are voiced).
7. *For discussion:* Most clinicians using a least knowledge method select to facilitate a new place or manner of production over a new voicing contrast. Interestingly, I do not recall ever having to decide in clinical practice between potential treatment targets that differed in the same number of place or manner features. To illustrate, in E's speech sample the choice is between [z] (which introduces a new manner of production) and [g] (which introduces a new place of production). Such a choice probably does not arise often in clinical care because the production capacity criterion limits the choice of possible treatment targets. For example, it is unlikely that E has any production capacity for [z]. Further, if E is able to produce both [g] and [z], most clinicians likely select both sounds for treatment rather than choose between them.

Answers for Exercise 15–4: Treatment Targets

1. **Words:** *pig, cat, door, fish, fan, cheese, house,* and *rabbit*
2. **Treatment targets:** The potential treatment targets are [p] in *pig*, [d] in *door*, [f] in *fish*, [tʃ] in *cheese*, [h] in *house*, and [æ] in *cat, fan,* and *rabbit.*
3. **Most or least knowledge:** a least knowledge method, because it affords more opportunities for generalization to occur
4. **Most knowledge and training deep:** There are at least two possible pairs of sounds. The first pair is [p] and [d], which share the same manner (stops) as many other consonants in Gavin's phonetic inventory. Both sounds also share the same places of production (bilabial and alveolar) as many other sounds in Gavin's phonetic inventory. Another possible pair is [f] and [p], which share the same voicing.
5. **Least knowledge and training wide:** There are at least two possible pairs of sounds. The first pair is [f] and [tʃ], which differ from each other in place and manner and also differ in place and manner from other sounds in Gavin's phonetic inventory. The other pair is [f] and [d], which differ from each other in place, manner, and voicing.
6. **Changing treatment targets (percentage):** Clients near Gavin's level of cognitive development (approximately 3 years of age) typically lack the cognitive and attention skills to perform well using a percentage criterion.
7. **Changing treatment targets:** Time offers structure to treatment while, at the same time, it somewhat replicates the gradual nature of acquisition. If the structure is too demanding for Gavin, a flexible criterion might also be attempted.
8. **Linguistic level (isolated sound or phrase):** Problems with use of isolated sounds include that they are not used outside the clinic (which makes generalization difficult) and they differ from what a client must do to speak, which more typically involves combining consonants and vowels. The problem with beginning at a phrase level with Gavin is that he has difficulty producing the treatment targets at the word level.
9. **Linguistic level:** The word level most closely approximates the skills Gavin uses outside the clinical setting.
10. **Phonetic environment:** The phonetic environment of treatment targets is the C in words with CV syllable structures.

Answers for Exercise 15–5: Treatment Targets

1. **Possible treatment targets**
   Stopping: [z] (*zoo*)
   [v] (*van, vest*)
2. **Possible treatment targets:**
   Gliding: [l] (*telescope, clown, balloon, Santa Claus, jelly, yellow, lamp, leaf, lion, elephant*)
   [r] (*train, radio, rain*)
   Cluster Reduction: [tʃr] (*train* is pronounced with an initial affricate in Kelly's dialect)
   [kl] (*clown, Santa Claus*)
   [nd mp nt] (nasal + stop) (*hand, lamp, elephant*)
   Affrication: [s] (*bus*)

3. **Summary of possible treatment targets:**
   Stopping: [z v]
   Gliding: [l r]
   Cluster Reduction: [tʃ r kl nd mp nt]
   Affrication: [s]
4. **Most or least knowledge:** The least knowledge method provides more opportunities for generalization. However, Kelly's speech is too developed for there to be only minimal differences between the two methods.
5. **Training wide or deep:** Training wide affords more opportunities for generalization.
6. **Changing treatment targets:** Time reflects the gradual nature of acquisition better than percentage and provides more structure than flexibility.
7. **Linguistic level:** The word level most closely approximates the skills Kelly uses outside the clinical setting.
8. **Phonetic environments:**
   Stopping: [z] word finally
   [v] word initially
   Gliding: [l] word initially, word medially in syllable initial position, and in word initial consonant clusters
   [r] word initially
   Cluster Reduction: [tʃr] word initially
   [kl] word initially
   [nd mp nt] (nasal + stop) word finally
   Affrication: [s] word finally

Answers for Exercise 15–6: Treatment Targets

1. **Selection technique:** phonetic placement (another possible answer is that Billy is stimulable for [r] at the level of the isolated sound)
2. **Most or least knowledge:** As Billy's speech contains so few errors, you need to select a most knowledge method. In fact, Billy's articulation and phonology is so sufficiently developed that no difference exists between the two methods.
3. **Training deep or wide:** The only option is to train deep, as only one sound is in error. However, if you selected to include [r] in consonant clusters in the short-term goal, a kind of training deep would have resulted if treatment included [r] in a variety of different consonant clusters.
4. **Changing treatment targets:** The only viable option is percentage, as the short-term goal includes only one sound. Most likely, given Billy's level of cognitive development and apparently intact attention abilities, a percentage criterion would be selected even if several sounds were receiving treatment. However, in the latter situation a time criterion might be used if Billy experienced cognitive or attention limitations.
5. **Linguistic level:** As Billy is stimulable for [r] at the word level, select that level to begin treatment. (Alternately, a clinician might select to first establish [r] as an isolated sound or in a short syllable.) After the sound is well established at the word level, the clinician would likely begin treatment at the phrase level.
6. **Phonetic environment:** Select word initial position. Although some clients appear to find [i] a facilitative vowel for [r], results of the speech sample and word probe do not suggest that this is the case for Billy. For this reason, begin treatment for [r] in the context of various vowels.

Answers for Exercise 16–1: Administrative Decisions

1. **Sessions:** Individual sessions often provide the quiet and freedom from distractions needed to introduce new treatment targets and to establish treatment routines. Group therapy, because it is a more natural setting involving other clients, is often preferred to help promote generalization and to maintain what has been learned.
2. **Session frequency:** Shorter treatment sessions may best mesh with the client's attention ability better than longer sessions, and more frequent sessions may keep the client more involved and focused on treatment than less frequent sessions.
3. **Length of sessions:** Individual sessions typically range from 10 or 15 minutes to 1 hour, and group sessions typically range from 30 to 45 minutes.
   Length of activities in sessions: Length of activities in sessions typical range from less than a minute to 30 minutes.
4. **Formats:** drill, drill play, structured play, and play

Answers for Exercise 16–2: Administrative Decisions

1. **Types of sessions:** Provide individual sessions early in treatment to help establish treatment routines and to introduce new treatment targets. As the treatment targets become established in Gavin's speech, most clinicians would likely begin to include targets in group sessions.
2. **Frequency of sessions:** Treatment sessions are likely scheduled from two to five times weekly. Given the severity of Gavin's articulation and phonological difficulties, most clinicians would likely select frequent sessions.
3. **Length of sessions:** Individual sessions typically last from 20 to 30 minutes and early intervention sessions typically last from 30 to 45 minutes.
4. **Length of activities:** Activities in treatment sessions typically last from a few minutes to 10 minutes.
5. **Format of activities:** Play is the most appropriate activity for Gavin's level of cognitive development. Another viable option is structured play.

Answers for Exercise 16–3: Administrative Decisions

1. **Types of sessions:** Provide individual sessions early in treatment to help establish treatment routines and to introduce new treatment targets. As the treatment targets become established, begin to include them in group sessions.
2. **Frequency of sessions:** Treatment sessions are scheduled from from two to five times weekly.
3. **Length of sessions:** Both individual and group sessions typically last from 30 to 45 minutes.
4. **Length of activities:** Activities in treatment session typically last up to 10 minutes.
5. **Format of activities:** Select structured play or drill play. Some research indicates that drill play is more effective and efficient than structured play with clients in Stage 3 and is equally as effective as drill (Shriberg & Kwiatowski, 1982).

Answers for Exercise 16–4: Administrative Decisions

1. **Types of sessions:** Provide individual sessions early in treatment to help establish [r] and then change to group sessions to help facilitate generalization to other settings.
2. **Frequency of sessions:** Treatment sessions typically occur from two to five times weekly. Because Billy's articulation and phonological disorder is not severe, most busy clinicians would likely opt for less frequent session scheduling.
3. **Length of sessions:** Individual sessions generally last from 30 to 45 minutes and early intervention sessions typically last from 45 minutes to 1 hour.
4. **Length of activities:** Activities in treatment sessions typically last from 10 to 15 minutes.
5. **Format of activities:** Most clinicians would typically select drill play and, possibly, some drill as well.

Answers for Exercise 17–1: Assessing Treatment Progress

1. **Pre- and posttests:** Two important types of pre- and posttests are word probes and judgment scales of severity and/or intelligibility.
2. **Number of words:** A general rule of thumb is 10 words per treatment target.
3. **Advantages:** Use of clinical judgment scales is time efficient. Further, they reflect important aspects of treatment— namely, degree of severity and intelligibility.
4. **Disadvantages:** Clinical judgment scales can be highly subjective. Also, scales that show only a few degrees of disability may not be sufficiently sensitive to detect smaller increments of improvement.
5. **Advantage:** Ongoing information gathering allows the clinician to monitor a client's treatment progress more closely.
6. **Disadvantage:** Ongoing information gathering can be time consuming and can direct attention away from the client during treatment sessions.

7. **Difference:** Single-subject design experiments allow the clinician to distinguish the effect of treatment from such variables as time and maturation. Other methods to assess treatment progress only serve to demonstrate whether or not a change occurs during treatment; such methods do not provide the clinician with unambiguous knowledge that a change is from treatment rather than other factors.

8. **[t] and [d]:** The sounds are closely related, making it likely that one will improve with treatment on the other.

9. *For discussion:* Typically, standardized assessment instruments only assess each sound a few times. Thus, if treatment results in improvement in only a few sounds, such change is not likely to appear significant using a standardized assessment instrument, even though it may represent a substantial gain for the client. To illustrate, suppose that in one semester a school-age client acquires [s] word initially, medially, and finally. A standardized test might cover 75 items, only three assessing [s]. In such a situation, the client's score only reflect improvement in three of 75 possible items in a semester, which is a small gain if the standardized test is used to assess treatment progress, even though the acquisition of [s] may represent a very important advance in development for the client.

Answers for Exercise 17–2: Assessing Treatment Progress

1. **Pretest:** One option is to use Tommy's initial speech sample as a pretest. Another option is to develop an error probe for Prevocalic Voicing. Concurrent with either method, a clinical judgment scale of severity or intelligibility might be administered.

2. **Pretest:** Prevocalic Voicing occurs 100% of the time. The words that undergoes Prevocalic Voicing are 1, 2, 5, 6, 7, and 11.

3. **Ongoing information gathering:** Treatment progress typically is assessed every session.

4. **Pre- and posttests:** Treatment progress is assessed at major junctions in treatment, such as every month, or the end of the semester, or after Tommy appears to have shown therapeutic gains.

5. **Posttest:** As with the pretest, the occurrence of Prevocalic Voicing is tabulated based on the words Tommy speaks during the final session. Alternately, you might develop a short (5- to-10 word) error probe as a posttest. Concurrent with either method, you might also administer a clinical judge scale of severity or intelligibility.

6. **Treatment effect:** Although likely the results of treatment, it also is possible that Tommy improved through maturation or through the efforts of someone else—perhaps a family member. There is more likelihood of treatment having been the agent of change if only Prevocalic Voicing, as only that error pattern received treatment.

7. **Assessment method:** single-subject design experiment (most likely a single-subject design across behaviors)

Answers for Exercise 17–3: Assessing Treatment Progress

1. **Pretest:** Determine the percentage of variability in Gavin's speech by dividing the number of variable words by the number of words produced without variability.

2. **Variability:** Of the 35 words, 13 words (37%) are produced with interword variability.

3. **Posttest:** The same words that receive treatment should be included in the posttest, because the goal of treatment is to reduce variability in certain specific words. For this reason, it is necessary that the words that receive treatment be included on both the pre- and posttests.

4. *For discussion:* The words being treated should be included in the pre- and posttests when the goal of treatment is to facilitate specific words. This often is the case with clients in Stage 2, but also occurs with clients in other stages who have difficulty with specific words. Illustrations of such situations include a child whose name begins with [l] being taught to pronounce [l] in his or her name, or an older child or an adult being taught to pronounce *astronomy* for his or her science class.

5. *For discussion:* Words being treated should not be included on the pre- and posttests when the treatment goal is to facilitate more general types of learning, which is typically the situation for many clients in Stage 2 and the vast majority of clients in Stages 3 and 4. To illustrate, most clients in Stage 3 are taught [k] in words such as *key* and *cough* not because these words are important in themselves, but because the words serve as vehicles whereby the client learns to pronounce [k] in all words that begin with [k] in the adult language. In such situations, the pre- and posttests demonstrate if generalization to other words has occurred.

Answers for Exercise 17–4: Assessing Treatment Progress

1. **Options:** The major options are to use the speech sample as a pretest or to develop short word probes for that purpose. Clinical judgment scales of severity or intelligibility might be performed in conjunction with either method.
2. **Error probe:** A possible error probe for Stopping in word initial position includes a range of fricatives before different vowels, such as *sign, feet, zoo, show, vine.*
3. **Error probe:** A possible error probe for Cluster Reduction in word initial position includes *drum, blue, spot, string, queen.*
4. **Treatment:** probably not, as Kelly's articulation and phonological difficulties involve sound classes rather than sounds in particular words
5. *For discussion:* Error probes are designed to fit the client's needs. If an error pattern occurs across a number of word positions, the pretest probe will need to be larger (perhaps 10 words). However, if the initial speech sample suggests that an error pattern only occurs in a single word position, the pretest may be shorter (perhaps 5 words).

Answers for Exercise 17–5: Assessing Treatment Progress

1. **Imitation:** Yes, the word probe can be used as a pretest, if you note the method of elicitation in the clinical report. However, as imitation is a fairly unnatural speech activity, most clinicians would likely want the pretest to include measures such as clinical judgment scales of severity or intelligibility.
2. **Clinical report:** Billy is able to produce word initial [r] in nonclusters 30% of the time during imitation.
3. **Posttest:** Most clinicians, myself included, prefer to use the same procedures for pre- and posttests. This way the clinician is comparing "apples to apples and oranges to oranges." If different methods are used in the pre- and posttests (for example, imitation in the pretest and sentence completion in the posttest), it is difficult to compare the two, as any changes in the client's speech might reflect differences in assessment methodology rather than the treatment, itself.
4. **Treatment result:** Although it seems likely that Billy's improvement results from treatment, you cannot entirely rule out the possibility that Billy's improvement results from such factors as maturation or the influence of a teacher or a family member. Such factors are not bad, of course—but they do make the results of treatment more difficult to demonstrate.

Answers for Exercise 18–1: Bombardment

1. **Fish book:** Present Ethan with a large colorful book about fish. Show Ethan pictures in the book, highlighting words containing [f], such as *fish, fins, fly* (for catching fish), *fishing boots,* and *fire* (for cooking fish).
2. **Baby book:** Show Ethan pictures in his favorite book about babies, highlighting body parts such as *fingers* and *feet,* and pointing out objects in the pictures such as *flowers, forks,* and *furry cats.*
3. **Cars and garage:** Set out a favorite toy car and a toy parking garage. While you and Ethan play, talk about the *fire engine,* the *Ford truck,* the *Firebird,* and the fffff sound of a leaky tire.
4. **Interactive play:** Engage Ethan in a game of "Where's the . . ." For this game, place objects around the room whose names contain the treatment target, and then, very energetically and playfully, ask Ethan questions such as, "Where's the frog?" When Ethan finds the frog, praise him, saying something like, "Yeah! You found the frog!" Then ask for the other objects, following the same procedure.
5. **Snack:** Help Ethan with his snack (or pretend snack, if no real snacks are available), emphasizing words such as *food, fingers* (for picking up food), *fork* (if applicable), *fruit,* and *fun.*
6. **ADL:** Help Ethan wash his face, emphasizing such words as *face* and *finger.* Make a game of cleaning the fingers, for each finger saying something like, "Now this finger."
7. *For discussion:* The rationale for providing bombardment for a client who appears temporarily stalled in development is to increase the frequency of the treatment target in the client's environment and, thus (hopefully) to facilitate the client's continued articulation and phonological development. I am not familiar with research on whether bombardment by itself has been shown to be an effective technique.

Answers for Exercise 18–2: Bombardment

1. **Stuffed animals:** Have stuffed animals tell Ethan stories that contain [k]. For example, a stuffed bear might tell a story about "A kangaroo who kicked the cough syrup off the cliff."
2. **Assorted toys:** During free play fill the room with toys including such things as *kangaroo, crayons,* and *castle.* Play with the toys, naming them frequently, and using facilitative talk techniques such as expansions, modeling, and parallel-talk.
3. **Cookie Monster:** Make a Cookie Monster face and attach it to a box in which a hole has been made for the mouth. Tell Tess that Cookie Monster is hungry and that he wants toys to eat. Name the toys one by one as Tess feeds them to Cookie Monster.
4. **Bean bag ball:** Mount pictures on the wall containing [k], such as *crab, cup,* and *crow.* Discuss a little with Tess about baseball. Tell her that she's the pitcher and that she is to pitch the ball to hit the pictures. Name the pictures as she hits them.
5. **Hide-and-seek:** Hide pictures or objects containing [k] around the room. Name the words, emphasizing the treatment target as Tess finds them.
6. **Lunch:** Ask Tess to bring her favorite doll or dolls to treatment. Arrange meal place settings and pretend that everyone is going out to lunch. During the course of play, talk and ask questions about such things as *cups, cola, cake, crackers,* and *cookies.*
7. **Quicker activity:** Perhaps the simplest bombardment activity is to read Tess a list of approximately 10 words containing the treatment target.
8. *For discussion:* The experience of many clinicians is that clients appear more focused on bombardment activities when such a system is used. The limitation of such a system, of course, is that its use requires a special room and equipment. In appropriate circumstances, any type of amplification system (such as are used in Karaoke toys) may offer a less expensive alternative to an FM frequency system.

Answers for Exercise 18–3: Bombardment

1. **Tongue twisters:** Recite tongue twisters containing [r]. An example of a possible tongue twister is, "The raging red river runs rapidly over old Red River Road."
2. **Poems or songs:** Proceed as with tongue twisters, except recite a poem or song containing many instances of [r], such as "The little red rooster comes bob bob bobbing along." (*Note:* If appropriate, extend the activity by having Billy draw a picture of the red rooster.)
3. **Blindfold:** Set objects containing [r] on a table. Blindfold Billy and tell him he is to find the object you name. Move the objects around and begin naming them for Billy to find when he hears each name.
4. **Naming cards:** The quickest form of this activity is for the clinician to name approximately 10 cards that contain [r]. An alternative activity is to show Billy 5 cards and then to place the cards face down on a table. Instruct Billy to turn over the card you name. Rename the card as he turns it over. After completing the first 5 cards, perform the same activity with the remaining 5 cards.
5. **Story:** Read Billy a story containing many words with [r]. The story might be one of Billy's favorites or one developed specifically for bombardment activities. If desired, instruct Billy to ring a bell, raise his hand, or clap his hands each time [r] occurs. (*Note:* An alternative activity is to read Billy a school lesson rather than a story, emphasizing [r] as it occurs.)

Answers for Exercise 19–1: Increasing Awareness

1. **Stages:** late Stage 3 and Stage 4
2. **Metaphors:**

Metaphors

Sound	Metaphors
[p]	Popping sound
[b]	Bubble sound
	Water boiling sound

(continued)

Metaphors *(continued)*

Sound	Metaphors
	Water jug sound
[t]	Tick-tock sound
[d]	Do sound ("I do it!")
	Homer Simpson sound (Doh!)
	Jackhammer sound
	Woodpecker sound
[k]	Cawing crow sound
	Coughing sound
[g]	Water pouring sound
	Baby babbling sound
	Frog sound
	"Great!" sound (Tony the Tiger sound)
[f]	Angry cat sound
[v]	Vacuum sweeper sound
	Housefly sound
	Jet sound
[θ]	Leaking tire sound
[ð]	Motor-on sound
[s]	Whistling teakettle sound
	Snake sound
	Hissing sound
[z]	Bee sound
[ʃ]	Hushing sound
	Quiet sound
	Seashell sound
[ʒ]	Motor sound
[tʃ]	Choo choo train sound
	Sneezing sound (choo!)
[dʒ]	Motor boat sound
[m]	Humming sound
	Taste good sound
	Spinning top sound
[n]	Mosquito sound
	Siren sound
[ŋ]	Electric wire sound
	Gong sound
[l]	Singing sound (la-la-la)
	Lullaby sound
[ɚ]	Mad dog sound (grrr)
	Growling tiger sound
	Arm wrestling sound
[r]	Dog woofing sound
	Starting race car sound
[j]	Yo-yo sound
	"Yes!" sound
[w]	"Wow!" sound
	Wind sound
[h]	Panting dog sound

Answers for Exercise 19–2: Increasing Awareness

1. **Cawing crow sound:** Show Tess a picture of a large black crow and imitate the cawing sound it makes. Talk about crows and their significance to a farmer, explaining how scarecrows are supposed to keep crows away from the farmer's fields by making them think the farmer is out working in his field. Next, read a story about a crow, finding opportunities to make "cawing" noises during the reading.

2. **Coughing sound:** Demonstrate a cough. Have Tess cough and ask her to think about where she feels the cough in her throat. Explain that this is the location where the [k] sound is made.

3. **Motor boat sound:** Bring in a small plastic boat and demonstrate the sound of the engine. Next, read Tess a story with a motor boat in the plot, taking advantage of all opportunities to make the motor boat sound.

4. **Whistling teakettle sound:** Bring in a teakettle and hot plate and allow Tess to listen to the whistling sound produced when air is allowed to escape through a small hole in the top of the teakettle. Tell Tess that the sound made by the teakettle is the whistling teakettle sound.

5. **Long sound:** Determine if Tess understands the concepts of *long* and *short* by asking her to select long and short objects from pairs of pencils, strings, rubber bands, and erasers. After you are certain that Tess understands the concept of *long*, engage Tess in alternately making long and short sounds while pulling tape out of a tape measure. For example, have Tess pull out the tape a considerable distance while producing [s] and a short distance while producing [t]. Continue having Tess produce long and short sounds using a variety of visual aids that can clearly be made long and short, such as elastic, rubber bands, and modeling clay.

6. **End sound:** Select pairs of identical toy objects for which "ends" can be distinguished, such as plastic dogs with and without tails, kites with and without kite tails, pencils with and without erasers, electrical cords with and without plugs, lollipop sticks with and without lollipops, or toothbrushes with and without rubber picks. Present each pair to Tess, asking her to identify whether the object has an end or not. Next, place all the objects together in the center of a table and ask Tess to separate the objects with an "end" from the objects without an "end."

7. **Sound friends:** Read Tess a story about friends. Explain at the end of the story that some sounds, like friends, like to be together. Give Tess examples of words containing sound friends (i.e., consonant clusters).

Answers for Exercise 19–3: Increasing Awareness

1. **Description of [s]:** "Do you remember when we listened to the teakettle whistle? The air had to come through the small hole so it would make a whistling sound. When you make the [s] sound, the air comes through a small hole between your teeth. Look in the mirror. Watch how I put my teeth together in the front. Do you see my tongue? No, you can't see my tongue. It is behind my front teeth. It stays out of the way so it doesn't block the hole. Now I will let some air come through the little hole between my front teeth. Put your hand in front of my mouth. You can feel the air coming through. Do you hear the whistling sound?"

2. **Lifesaver:** Tie a length of dental floss onto a lifesaver. Ask Kelly to place her tongue into the hole of the lifesaver and hold it against the alveolar ridge behind the upper front teeth. Tell Kelly that this is where she is to place her tongue when making the "whistling teakettle" ([s]) sound.

3. **Tongue lowered:** The lifesaver would be placed behind the lower front teeth.

4. **Chewing gum:** Sit with Kelly in front of a mirror, both of you chewing sugar-free gum. Demonstrate to Kelly how to hold the gum up behind her teeth on the gum ridge with her tongue. If Kelly is unable to hold the gum in this position, put on latex gloves and place her chewing gum on her alveolar ridge and have her hold it in this position with her tongue. (*Note:* To make the activity more fun, have a contest to see who can hold the chewing gum in place the longest when the mouth is open and only the elevated tongue tip holds the gum to the alveolar ridge.)

5. **Ticking clock:** Tell Kelly to make a noise like a clock that goes tick-tick-tick-tick-tick. Ask her to note the place where her tongue touches the roof of her mouth behind her top teeth. Tell her that this is where her tongue tip needs to be when producing the [s] sound. (*Note:* If desired, follow up on this activity by helping Kelly draw a picture showing an open mouth with the tongue raised to the alveolar ridge.)

6. **Tongue depressor and mirror:** Sit with Kelly before a mirror. Demonstrate touching your alveolar ridge with your tongue. Insert a tongue depressor or cotton swab between your alveolar ridge and your tongue and breathe out. Tell Kelly that is how the air should sound when she makes an [s]. After completing the demonstration on yourself, perform the same demonstration with Kelly.

7. **Manner of production:** Ask Kelly to put her teeth together gently, to raise her tongue up to the ridge behind her front teeth, to smile, and breathe in, and then to gently blow air out. If needed, remind Kelly to make the "whistling teakettle" sound.

8. **[t] to [s]:** Ask Kelly to make [t] several times. Contrast the shortness of [t] with sounds like [s] and [h], which can be "held out." Have a contest to see who can hold out various continuant sounds the longest. Next, ask Kelly to make a [t] sound and to "hold it out." (*Note:* For some clients this simple demonstration by itself is successful in facilitating their acquisition of [s].)

Answers for Exercise 20–1: Facilitating Syllables and Words

1. **Principle:** The basic principle underlying word pairs is that languages use sounds to distinguish between the meaning of words.

2. **Stages:** Word pairs are most appropriate for more cognitively advanced clients in Stage 3 and clients in Stage 4.

3. **Bean bag toss:** Place large picture cards representing word pairs such as *bus/bum* on the floor at least 18" apart. To verify that Tess knows the words, ask her to name the pictures. Ignore incorrect pronunciations and either select new pictures or teach the vocabulary for the pictures she cannot name. Instruct Tess to throw a bean bag onto each picture named by the examiner. Otherwise, tape picture pairs (such as *bus/bum*) on the wall, asking Tess to use the bean bag to hit each word named.

4. **Barrier game:** Sit across the table from Tess with a barrier between you. Have one set of pictures of paired words before Tess on her side of the table and a duplicate set before you. Ask Tess to hold up cards as you name them. After each of Tess' responses, pick up the card from your set that Tess named to either confirm or negate her answer. (*Note:* Vary the number of cards in view at one time depending on the client's age, cognitive level, and attention span.)

5. **Fishing game:** Create a fishing pole with a ruler or pencil as a rod, string for line, and a small magnet for a hook. Place Tess on one side of a barrier with paired word cards before her, each having an attached paper clip to adhere to the magnet on the fishing pole. You fish from the other side of the barrier, naming the cards for which you are fishing. Instruct Tess to select the card you name and to attach it to the fishing line.

6. **Magic box:** Create a magic box containing objects representing paired words. Ask Tess to reach into the box, feel the objects, and bring out the object named by the examiner.

7. **Puppets:** Introduce Tess to the puppets, explaining that Tess' job is to help the puppet who has trouble speaking. For example, during a walk through the jungle one of the puppets might instruct the others to listen because snakes *hit* before they strike. If needed, prompt Tess to tell the puppet that snakes *hiss* before they strike. (*Note:* Many times, children particularly enjoy the "sillier" mistakes of the puppet.)

8. **Goat:** Tell Tess a story about goats and their eating habits. Afterwards, make a goat out of a small box. Explain to Tess that this goat, although eating many "weird" things, has some picky eating habits. For example, the goat only eats things whose words begin with [r]. Place pictures of word pairs on a table and ask Tess which word the goat wants to eat. To illustrate, place pictures of *wing* and *ring* on the table, asking Tess to identify which picture the goat won't eat. After Tess identifies *wing*, ask Tess to say *ring* so that the goat will eat it. Place the *ring* card in the goat box when Tess says it with an initial [r]. Otherwise, have Tess feed it to the goat.

Answers for Exercise 20–2: Facilitating Syllables and Words

1. **Reading aloud:** Show Billy a picture while reading aloud a passage that lacks one word. Provide Billy pictures of a word pair, asking him to point to the word that belongs in the sentence. For example, the passage might be, "The lookout point is dangerous. That's why they built a _____." The word pair is *rail* and *whale*. (*Note:* This activity can be adapted for an older client by not having pictures and asking the client write his or her answer on an answer sheet.)

2. **Bingo:** Use word pair picture cards in a Bingo Game, explaining to Billy that he is to put a token on each word you name. Place word pairs under the same column so Billy must make distinctions between them. For example, under "I" place *reed* and *weed*, and call out "I - reed," making Billy distinguish between [w] and [r] to place the token correctly.

3. **Story:** Read Billy a story, instructing him to raise his hand every time the story contains a word pronounced incorrectly. For example, a sentence in the story might be, "It was a beautiful wed apple." (*Note:* This activity can be adapted for older clients by reading a school assignment instead of a story.)

4. **Board game:** Play a board game appropriate for a client in a lower elementary grade, such as tic-tac-toe, Connect-Four, Battleship, or Go Fish. Instruct Billy that prior to each turn he must answer a question that requires him to pronounce one member of a word pair for a statement to make sense. An example of such a question is, "Do clothes with a tear have a rip or a whip?" Billy is then required to answer, "Rip." (*Note:* This activity can be adapted for older clients by deleting the game and simply asking the client to answer questions. For example, "Do you go skating at a rink or a wink?")

5. **Billiards:** Tape photocopied pictures of word pairs to the sides of each pocket of a tabletop billiards game. Tell Billy each word is the name of one of the pockets. For example, the first pocket is named *wing*, the second is named *ring*, the third is named *red*, and fourth is named *wed*. The rule of the game is that Billy must call out the pocket for which he is aiming. Award points if Billy gets the ball into the pocket he named.

6. **Barrier game:** Set out identical objects or pictures on both sides of the barrier. These should represent common household items such as a table, bed, chair, and rug (a colored piece of paper). Explain to Billy that these "rooms" (each side of the barrier) belong to some messy kids and that Billy is the parent. Billy's job is to tell the kids how to clean up their rooms so that the two rooms look exactly alike. For example, Billy might say, "Put the ring under the table. Put the radio on the table. Put the chair by the rug."

Answers for Exercise 20–3: Facilitating Syllables and Words

1. **Chalkboard:** Ask Tess to stand at a chalkboard. Instruct her to prolong the vowel in words as she draws a line. When Tess runs out of room at the edge of the chalkboard, tell her she must put on the "end" of the word (the final consonant). For example, for *big* Tess says "biiiiiiiiiiiiiiiiiii," and then adds [g] when she runs out of chalkboard. (*Note:* If the client is unable to perform the activity independently after several models, the clinician may want to produce several words simultaneously with the client.)

2. **Snake:** Work with Tess to establish the "hissing sound" as metaphor for [s]. Using a rubber snake, take turns with Tess helping the snake say s-s-s-s-s-s. Place objects on the table whose names can be preceded by [s] to form another word. Examples of possible objects include *pin* (to make *spin*) and *nail* (to make *snail*). Tell Tess that every time the snake tries to say a word an [s] sound is put in front of the word. Demonstrate this by using the objects on the table (i.e., the snake says *pin* as *spin*). Ask Tess if she can say the words like the snake does.

3. **Clapping or tapping:** Read multisyllabic words to Tess, asking her to clap her hands or tap her feet for each syllable. If needed, begin with two-syllable words before attempting longer words.

4. **Production:** Ask Tess to pronounce a list of multisyllabic words, saying each syllable with equal intensity and duration, clapping her hand or tapping her foot for each syllable. For example, Tess would pronounce both *money* and *below* as STRONG-STRONG. After Tess masters this task, ask her to clap her hands or tap her feet while pronouncing the same words, alternating loud-soft and short-long syllables. Next, introduce a key word and rhythm cue such as "the elephant's beat" for words such as *telephone* that have STRONG-weak-strong stress patterns. Continue to provide Tess practice in pronouncing words with "the elephant's beat," using hand clapping or foot tapping as needed.

5. **Other syllable retention activities:** Among the many possible ways of indicating syllables in words are clicking a clicker, buzzing a buzzer, ringing a bell, striking a triangle, beating a drum, hitting a key on a xylophone, or dropping objects into a container.

6. **Spinning wheel game:** Make a spinning wheel containing pictures of things that can contain an [r] to form a new word. For example the wheel might contain *diver* (to make *driver*), *bed* (to make *bread*), *room* (to make *broom*), and *root* (to make *fruit*). Place a spinner in the middle of the wheel and a large "r" at the top of a chalkboard to which the spinning wheel is attached. Ask Billy to spin the wheel. Each time the wheel stops at a word, ask Billy what new word is made if an [r] is added right after the first sound. If the goal of the activity is to facilitate perception, Billy might indicate which new word is formed by picking an appropriate picture. Production might be facilitated by asking Billy to name the new word.

7. **Connect-the-dots:** As with Tess, use perception and production activities involving words with equal and alternating syllable lengths and intensities, key words, and rhythm cues. For the perception activities, ask Billy to draw a line to connect dots for each syllable he hears. For the production activities, ask Billy to retrace the lines between dots for each syllable he says.

8. **Other syllable retention activities:** Among the many possible ways to indicate syllables in words are building a tower with one block for each syllable, tapping out syllables heard or spoken with an eraser of a pencil, or moving the number of spaces on a gameboard corresponding to the number of syllables heard or spoken.

Answers for Exercise 21–1: Indirect and Direct Techniques

1. **Stages:** Stage 2 and 3
2. **Facilitative talk:** Clients in Stage 2 and 3 often are unable to understand and follow direct instruction techniques.
3. **Facilitative talk:** modeling
4. **Facilitative talk:** requests for confirmation or clarification
5. **Facilitative talk:** parallel talk
6. **Facilitative talk:** motherese
7. **Facilitative talk:** expansion
8. **Facilitative talk:** strategic errors
9. *For discussion:* Facilitative talk serves as a type of "speech lesson" for the client. The "lesson" is achieved by simplifying the speech to which the client is exposed.

Answers for Exercise 21–2: Indirect and Direct techniques

1. **Bus activity:** Ask Matt if he wants to play. Bring out a toy garage, cars, and a bus. Place the bus toy near you and ask Matt to tell you which toys he wants. When Matt says *bus* as "ba," expand his utterance to "bus" or something like, "Here's the bus."
2. **Cake activity:** Set out toys that include a toy cake and a toy gate. As part of the activity, ask Matt which toy he wants. When Matt says [g] for *cake*, either say something like, "Do you want the gate?" or "Did you say you wanted the gate?" (request for confirmation).
3. **Parallel talk activity:** One of many possibilities is to fill a "Feely-Meely Box" with objects whose names end with a consonant. Ask Matt to name each object as he or you pull it from the box. Name the objects as Matt pulls them from the box, emphasizing the final consonant in each word.
4. **Telephone activity:** Set up a table and chairs and have Matt "telephone" to invite friends over to play (stuffed animals large enough to sit on child-size chairs at a small table). Use motherese by having the animals speak in a slightly higher than normal pitch and by using repetitions and exaggerated intonation. Use expansion by filling in missing sounds and syllables in the telephone conversation. Use requests for confirmation or clarification when Matt mispronounces a treatment target.
5. **Puppet activity:** Introduce Matt to a puppet who "wants to be Matt's friend." You hold the puppet and speak for it, making errors similar to those made by Matt. Use strategic errors and expansion with the puppet as well, so Matt sees that others also make mistakes. Use modeling techniques by asking the puppet and then Matt to answer questions. For example, if a goal of treatment is to facilitate word final consonants, show the puppet a toy dog, asking, "Want do?" Then say something like, "Matt—do you want a do*g*?"
6. **Arts and craft activity:** Bring out objects for an arts and craft activity. While Matt plays, engage in parallel talk about his actions. For example, if the goal is to facilitate Matt's acquisition of word final consonants, the clinician might say something like, "Ma*tt* is putting his han*d* in the glue po*t*." If Matt omits word final consonants when he speaks, expand his utterances, stressing the final consonants.

Answers for Exercise 21–3: Talking with Clients

1. **Clients:** more cognitively advanced clients in late Stage 3 and for most clients in Stage 4
2. **Phonetic placement and shaping:** Phonetic placement involves the physical placement of the client's articulators into position for production of the target sound. Shaping techniques involve a series of successive approximations from a sound in the client's repertoire to a target production.
3. **Snake activity:** Show Kelly pictures of a snake to demonstrate how quickly a snake can move its tongue in and out of its mouth. Next, review the metaphor lesson for [s] as the "hissing" sound, using a snake puppet (preferably one with a tongue) to make hissing noises with its tongue out. Have a "mother" snake tell the other snake(s) that, "it is not polite to stick out your tongue when you are talking to someone." Have the puppet snake continue to try hissing with its tongue inside while talking to Kelly. Next, have Kelly "hiss" with her tongue out. Instruct Kelly to slowly pull her tongue back inside her mouth while continuing to "hiss" softly. The [s] sound should result.

4. **Balloon activity:** Blow up a strong mylar balloon. Next, allow a slow leak in the balloon and have Kelly feel the air escaping. Hold the leaky spot to Kelly's ear for her to hear the air escaping. Next, tell Kelly to pretend that her mouth is a balloon and to suck air in slowly through her lightly closed teeth and to hold the air inside, not allowing any to escape. Then, take a small instrument and pretend to make a tiny hole in the front of Kelly's "balloon" between her closed front teeth. Instruct Kelly to let the air leak out slowly and steadily from between her front teeth. An [s] sound should result. (*Note:* After completing this activity, many children enjoy changing places with the clinician, making a leak in the clinician's balloon.)

5. **Teakettle activity:** First, review the metaphor for [s] as the teakettle sound with the client. Next, have the client pretend to be a teakettle with lots of steam inside. Have the client pretend that the slight opening between his or her closed teeth is the hole in the lid of the teakettle. Pretend to turn up the heat under the teakettle so that it gets hot. Tell the client to gradually allow steam (air) to escape through the opening in his or her lightly closed teeth. If needed, instruct the client to make the sound whistle. (*Note:* If the sound is "muffled" because the tongue rests too far forward, tell the client to slowly bring the tongue up and back and let it touch on the "little shelf" behind the top teeth (or on the ridge below the bottom teeth) to make the teakettle whistle.)

6. **Straw activity:** Begin by having Kelly pretend to be a space scientist who uses precise instrumentation (a soda straw) to select a target and to launch a missile. Next, place a straw between Kelly's lightly closed central incisors. Tell Kelly that to score a "hit," the air must be directed through the straw to hit the target. To help Kelly develop self-monitoring skills, instruct her to listen for the rush of air when it is successfully directed down the straw. An [s]-like sound with central air emission should result as Kelly "hits" the targets. (*Note:* To make the game more competitive, give Kelly a point for each "hit" and give yourself a point for each of the client's "misses.")

7. **Pocahontas activity:** Show Kelly a picture of a canoe, talking about how the canoe's sides are shaped. Next, let Kelly be Pocahontas canoeing in white water. Tell her she is a scout in the lead canoe and that her tribe is following behind her in other canoes. Pocahontas' job is to lead the way and to warn the others about upcoming dangers with a whistling sound ([s]), a secret signal known only to her tribe. Tell Kelly that to produce the secret signal, she will need to let the breathstream move down the middle of the tongue groove so that it makes a soft whistling sound as it passes the teeth. As part of this explanation, tell Kelly that her tongue is like a canoe and that the sides of the tongue must be kept up so that water will not come in and tip the canoe. An [s] should result as Kelly attempts to warn the tribe of dangers along the river.

8. **Woodpecker activity:** Show Kelly a picture of a woodpecker and talk to her about how the woodpecker pecks holes in wood, demonstrating the woodpecker sound as a rapid succession of t-t-t-t-t-t. Ask Kelly to imitate the woodpecker sound, making the t-t-t-t-t-t as rapidly as possible. As part of this activity, have a contest with Kelly to see who can repeat t-t-t-t-t-t the longest without taking a breath. Afterwards, talk about how tired the tongue gets making this sound in rapid succession. Next, tell Kelly to make the woodpecker sound again. After Kelly makes a few woodpecker sounds in rapid succession, tell her that when the woodpecker gets tired his tongue rests up on the shelf behind the top teeth, but that his breath continues to come out. Talk Kelly through this scenario until [s] is produced.

9. **Jackhammer activity:** Explain to Kelly what a jackhammer does. Ask her to pretend she is a jackhammer by rapidly repeating t-t-t-t-t-t. Next, tell Kelly to make the sound again and to pretend the motor got "stuck" on [t]. Tell Kelly to keep her motor running, but to keep her tongue stuck on [t] by resting it on the shelf behind her top teeth. Keep playing until [s] results.

APPENDIX
B

Longer Speech Samples From Children Developing Typically

APPENDIX B–1

Hildegard

BACKGROUND: Hildegard is 2 years, 0 months of age, is being raised bilingually (German and American English), and speaks a variety of midwestern English (Leopold, 1947).

Reliability

The reliability measures of the published studies and transcriptions are described in the original sources. Reliability tests were performed on approximately 10% of the speech in the unpublished studies. Inter- and intra-judge reliability of the phonetic transcriptions of the unpublished studies was at least 90% for consonants, vowels, stress patterns, syllable boundaries, and diacritics. The diacritics are those described in Chapter 2 of Bleile (1995).

WORD LIST

Intended Words	Hildegard	Intended Words	Hildegard	Intended Words	Hildegard
1. pillow	bi	47. beach	bitʃ	94. New York	nɔjɔk
2. piece	bis	48. boy	bɔɪ	95. nose	nos
3. peas	bi	49. bug	bok	96. new	nu
4. piano	ba	50. book	bok	97. forgot	dat
5. papa	baba	51. boot	bot	98. feed	wi
6. pail	be.a	52. boat	bot	99. feet	wit
7. pick	bɪt	53. balloon	bu	100. fix	wɪt
8. put	bʊ	54. broken	bok	101. fall	wɔ
9. paper	bubu	55. brief	bitʃ	102. fork	wɔk
10. pudding	bʊ.ɪ	56. blow	bo	103. fly	waɪ
11. push	bʊʃ	57. block	bak	104. flower	waʊ
12. poor	pu	58. down	dɔ	105. Florence	woʃ
13. pretty	pɪti	59. dolly	da.i	106. throw	do
14. please	bis	60. duck	dak	107. through	tu
15. towel	daʊ	61. dear	diə	108. three	wi
16. toast	dok	62. door	do	119. soap	haʊx
17. too	du	63. Dodo	dɔdɔ	110. sandbox	jabak
18. toothbrush	tuʃbaʃ	64. don't	dot	111. slide	jaɪ
19. two	tu	65. doggie	doti	112. spoon	bu
20. train	te	66. do	du	113. sticky	titi
21. cover	da	67. dry	daɪ	114. stocking	dadi
22. candy	da.i	68. drink	dɪk	115. stick	dɪk
23. kiss	dɪʃ	69. dress	daʃ	116. stone	dɔɪʃ
24. cold	do	70. go	do	117. scratch	daʃ
25. comb	do	71. gone	gɔ	118. shoe	ʒu
26. coat	dot~	72. Grandpa	ŋæŋæ	119. this	dɪt
	nʊk	73. man	ma	120. chicken	dɪkə
27. cake	gek	74. mine	maɪ	121. Joey	do.i
28. cookies	tutiʃ	75. money	maɪ	122. juice	du
29. cry	daɪ	76. mama	mama	123. highchair	aɪta
30. crash	daʃ	77. much	ma	124. hand	hã
31. cracker	gaga	78. mouse	maʊʃ	125. high	haɪ
32. buggy	baɪ	79. mouth	maʊʃ	126. Hildegard	haɪta
33. bike	baɪk	80. make	mek	127. Helen	haja
34. bite	baɪt	81. me	mi	128. hot	hat
35. box	bak	82. milk	mik	129. hat	hat
36. back	bakə	83. meat	mit	130. house	haʊs
37. bottle	bʌlu	84. Milwaukee	wati	131. hair	hea
38. ball	baʊ	85. now	na	132. here	hɪ
39. bell	baʊ	86. nice	naɪʃ	133. home	hɔ
40. bear	bea	87. night	naɪt	134. hello	jojo
41. baby	bebi	88. not	nat	135. water	walu
42. bake	bek	89. knee	ni	136. wash	waʃ
43. bacon	bekə	90. neck	nɪk	137. watch	waʃ
44. bathe	beʃ	91. no	nɔ	138. way	we
45. big	bi	92. naughty	nɔ.i	139. where	we
46. beads	bitʃ	93. noise	nɔɪs	140. wet	wet

WORD LIST

Intended Words	Hildegard	Intended Words	Hildegard	Intended Words	Hildegard
141. wait	wɛt	152. light	haɪt	163. auto	ʔaʊto
142. wheel	wi	153. lie	jaɪ	164. out	ʔaʊx
143. walk	wɔk	154. all	ʔa	165. airplane	ʔeɪpi
144. ride	haɪ	155. on	ʔa	166. egg	ʔɛk
145. room	hu	156. alley	ʔa.i	167. in	ʔɛt
146. write	jaɪ	157. egg	ʔaɪ	168. away	ʔəwe
147. right	waɪt	158. eye	ʔaɪ	169. ear	ʔi
148. read	wi	159. I	ʔaɪ	170. eat	ʔit
149. rug	wi	160. ironing	ʔaɪni	171. oil	ʔɔɪdo
150. Rita	wiwi	161. up	ʔap		
151. roll	wɔ	162. apple	ʔapa		

APPENDIX B–2

Kylie

BACKGROUND: Kylie is 2 years, 0 months of age and speaks a variety of midwestern English (Bleile, 1987).

WORD LIST

Intended Words	Kylie	Intended Words	Kylie	Intended Words	Kylie
1. puppy	pʌpi	26. Corrie	tɔwi	51. bible class	baɪbə bæs
2. puzzle	pʌzʊ	27. curtain	tʊ.ɪn	52. bed	bɛd
3. pony	poʊni	28. carrot	tɛwɪ	53. bee	bi
4. pear	pɛ	29. coming (v)*	tʌmɪn	54. balloon	bəlun
5. Teddy (Bear)	tɛdi	30. keys	tiz	55. balloons	bəlunz
6. turtle	tɝɾʊ	31. cake	teɪk	56. bathroom	bæθwum
7. tea	ti	32. corn	pɔn	57. bug	bʌg
8. table	teɪbʊ	33. cards	taɪz	58. blue	bəlu
9. two	toʊ	34. crying	baɪ.ɪn	59. break	beɪk
10. tired	taɪ.əd	35. cream	kwim	60. broken	boʊkɪn
11. too much	tu mʌts	36. clown	taʊn	61. bread	bwɛ
12. truck	bʌk	37. close	toʊz	62. duck	dʌk
13. tractor	bʌtsə	38. closed	toʊzd	63. ducks	dʌks
14. tree	bwi	39. Cliford	tɪfʊ	64. daddy	dædi
15. triangle	baɪ.æŋgʊ	40. quilt	pɪ	65. dog	dɔg
16. kitty	tɪɾi	41. queen	bwi	66. doggie	dɔgi
17. kitty cat	tɪtæ	42. baby	beɪbi	67. daisy	deɪzi
18. cow	taʊ	43. bear	bɛr	68. dolly	dɑdi
19. Cookie Monster	tʊɾi mɑnstə	44. bird	bʊd	69. go	doʊ
20. cookie	tʊki	45. birdie	bʊdi	70. girl	dʊ
21. Ken	tɛn	46. ball	bɔ	71. Grandpa	dæpə
22. coat	toʊ	47. book	bʊk	72. grapes	deɪps
23. car	tɑ	48. back (n)	bæk	73. grass	bwæs
24. candy	tæni	49. butterfly	bʌɾəfaɪ	74. green	bin
25. kiss	tɪs	50. bananas	bənænəs	75. Grab Bag Party	bɑbæg pɑɾi

(continued)

WORD LIST *(continued)*

Intended Words	Kylie	Intended Words	Kylie	Intended Words	Kylie
76. glasses	dæsɪz	119. seal	sid	162. highchair	haɪtɛ
77. mine	maɪn	120. Sarah	sɛwə	163. hungry	hʌŋgwi
78. me	mi	121. sock (n)	sɑk	164. why	waɪ
79. momma	mɑmɑ	122. socks	sɑks	165. watch (n)	wɑs
80. more	mɔ	123. Slinky	sɪŋki	166. walking	wɔkɪn
81. mouse	maʊs	124. sleeping	tipɪn	167. woops	wʊps
82. milk	mɛk	125. slide (n)	saɪd	168. yep	jɛp
83. monkey	mʌŋki	126. swimming suit	sumɪn sut	169. yah ([jæ])	jæ
84. messing (v)	mɛsɪn	127. sweater	bwɛzə	170. yogurt	joʊgʊt
85. mackerel	mækʊ	128. spider	spaɪdə	171. lion	jaɪ.ɪn
86. Mark	mʌk	129. spoon	spun	172. lamby	læmi
87. money	mʌni	130. spring	spwɪŋ	173. leg	jɛg
88. moon	mun	131. stars	stɑz	174. lawnmower	jæmaʊ
89. music	muzɪk	132. stops	stɑps	175. robin	wɑbɪn
90. man	mæn	133. stopped	stɑpt	176. read	wi
91. mens (pl)	mɛn	134. strawberries	stʌmbɛwiz	177. rabbit	wæbɪt
92. moo	mu	135. scare	stɛ	178. rabbits	wæbɪs
93. nest	nɛt	136. school	stʊ	179. raccoon	wækun
94. nose	noʊz	137. speaker	spikʊ	180. ring	wɪŋ
95. no	noʊ	138. snack	sneɪk	181. rock (n)	wɑk
96. nope	noʊp	139. snow	snoʊ	182. Amy	eɪmi
97. neck	nʌk	140. Snow White	snoʊ waɪt	183. airplane	oʊpweɪn
98. knee	ni	141. shovel	ʌvʊ	184. elephant	ɛfɪn
99. knife	naɪf	142. this	θɪs	185. apple	æpʊ
100. foot	fʊʔ	143. thanks	dæŋks	186. alright	ɔwaɪʔ
101. foots	fʊts	144. zebra	zɛbə	187. off	ɔf
102. fish (n)	fɛs	145. xenophone	zʌdəfoʊn	188. ok	oʊteɪ
103. fun	fʌn	146. chicken	tɪkɪn	189. upside down	ʌpsaɪdaʊn
104. first	fʊst	147. chickens	tɪkɪns	190. eye	aɪ
105. firemen	faɪ.əmɛn	148. cheeks	tiks	191. eyes	aɪz
106. frog	fɔg	149. jelly	dɛdi	192. ear	ir
107. flower	faʊwə	150. jumps	dʌmps	193. ears	ɛrz
108. flowers	faʊwəz	151. Jessie	dɛsi	194. ice cream	aɪs kwim
109. fly (n)	faɪ	152. jumping bean	dʌpə bin	195. owl	aʊwə
110. sad	sæd	153. (grass)hopper	hɑpə	196. on	ɑn
111. scissors	sɪzʊs	154. here	hir	197. umbrella	babɛwə
112. sidewalk	saɪwɔk	155. hands	hænz	198. again	ədɛn
113. sun	sʌn	156. hog	hɔg	199. outside	aʊsaɪd
114. sunglasses	tunbæsɪs	157. house	haʊs	200. open	oʊpɪn
115. circle	sɛkʊ	158. hamster	hæpstə	201. opens	oʊpɪnz
116. circles	sɛkʊs	159. hurt	hʊt	202. ouch	aʊ
117. cereal	sɪwɪ.ə	160. hair	hɛr	203. oops	ʊps
118. cereals	sɛwəs	161. happy	hapi		

* = In this and the following transcripts, v = verb, n = noun, and pl = plural.

APPENDIX B–3

Amahl

BACKGROUND: Amahl is 2 years, 0 months of age (Smith, 1973). Amahl's parents are English and Indian, and Amahl speaks a variety of British English.

WORD LIST

Intended Words	Amahl	Intended Words	Amahl	Intended Words	Amahl
1. park	bak	40. crying	gaɪ.ɪn	79. Granna	læla
2. pedal	pɛgʊ	41. baby	bebi	80. grape	geɪp
3. peg	pɛk	42. back	bɛk	81. greedy	gidi
4. pen	bɛn	43. ball	bɔ.	82. man	mæn~
5. penis	bɪnɪn	44. banana	banə		mɛn
6. pip	bɪp	45. bath	bat	83. men	mæn~
7. play	beɪ	46. bead	bit~		mɛn
8. please	bi		bid	84. mend	mɛn
9. table	bebʊ	47. beetle	bigʊ	85. Mike	maɪk
10. taking	geɪkɪn	48. bell	bɛ	86. milk	mɪk
11. taxi	gægi	49. better	bɛdə	87. mixer	mɪgə
12. teeth	tiθ	50. bird	bɪbip	88. moon	mu~
13. telephone	dɛwibu~	51. biscuit	bɪgi~		mun
	dɛwibun		bɪgɪk	89. more	mɔ
14. tent	dɛt	52. bit (n)	bɪt	90. motorcar	mugəga
15. tickle	gɪgʊ	53. bolt	bɔt	91. mice	maɪt
16. tie	daɪ	54. book	bʊk	92. knee	ni
17. tiger	gaɪgə	55. bottle	bɔgʊ	93. knife	maɪp
18. tongue	gʌŋ	56. bottom	bɔdɪn	94. naughty	nɔdi
19. turn	dʌn	57. boy	bɔɪ	95. new	nu
20. troddler	lɔlə	58. bump	bʌp	96. nice	naɪt
21. trolly	lɔli	59. burn	bʌn	96. nice	naɪt
22. trowel	daʊ	60. bus	bʌt	97. nipple	mɪbʊ
23. truck	gʌk	61. butterfly	bʌdəwaɪ	98. noisy	nɔni
24. cake	gek	62. black	bæk	99. nose	nu
25. caravan	gæwəwæn~	63. blow (v)	bu	100. now	naʊ
	gæwəvæn	64. broken	bʊgu	101. nut	nʌt
26. carpet	gabɪ	65. briefcase	bik keɪk	102. feet	wit
27. cat	mi.aʊ	66. brush (n/v)	bʌt	103. finger	wiŋə
28. coach	guk	67. Daddy	dɛdi	104. fire	wæ
29. cock	gɔk	68. dark	gak	105. follow	wɔwu
30. come	gʌm	69. ding-dong	gɪŋ gɔŋ	106. foot	wʊt
31. come out	gʌmaʊt	70. dog(ie)	wowo	107. fork	wɔk
32. corner	gɔnə	71. door	dɔ	108. thank-you	gɛgu
33. corridor	gɔɪdə	72. duck	gʌk	109. soap	up
34. cupboard	gʌbə	73. drink	gɪk	110. seat	it
35. curtain	gʌgən	74. driving	waɪbɪn	111. side	daɪt
36. key	gi	75. drum	dʌm	112. singing	gɪŋɪŋ
37. kiss	gɪk	76. dry	daɪ	113. scissors	dɪdə
38. crib	gɪb	77. good	gʊg	114. sock	gɔk
39. crumb	gʌm	78. glasses	gagi	115. soon	dun

(continued)

WORD LIST *(continued)*

Intended Words	Amahl	Intended Words	Amahl	Intended Words	Amahl
116. soup	up	149. juice	dut	184. lie (down)	daɪ daʊn
117. sunshine	dʌn daɪn~	150. hair	ɛ	185. light	daɪt
	ʌn daɪn	151. hammer	ɛmə	186. like	gaɪk
118. slipper	bɪbə	152. hand	ɛn	187. little	dɪdi
119. swing	wɪŋ	153. handle	ɛnu	188. lock	gɔk
120. switch	wɪt	154. hard	at	189. lolly (pop)	ɔli
121. spanner	bænə	155. head	ɛd	190. lorry	lɔli
122. spoon	bun	156. hello	ɛlu	191. lotion	dudən
123. sport	bɔt	157. home	um	192. rain	deɪn
124. stalk	gɔk	158. hot	ɔt	193. red	dɛt
125. stamp	dæp	159. house	aʊt	194. ring	gɪŋ
126. stuck	gʌk	160. hurt	ʌt	195. Robbie	wɔbi
127. sticky	gɪgi	161. one	wʌn	196. room	wʊm
128. stop	bɔp~	162. wash	wɔt	197. round	daʊn
	dɔp	163. watch	wɔt	198. rubber	bʌbə
129. struck	gok	164. wet	wɛt	199. rubberband	bʌbəbæn
130. stroke	gok	165. wheel	wi	200. running	dʌnin
131. sky	gaɪ	166. wheelbarrow	wibæwu	201. aeroplane	ɛbəʔeɪn
132. scream	gim	167. whistle	wɪbʊ~	202. angry	ɛŋi
133. screw	gu		wɪpʊ	203. ant	ɛt
134. smell	mɛn	168. window	wɪnu	204. Adrian	edi
135. Smith	mɪt	169. working	wʌgɪn	205. apple	ɛbʊ
136. snake	neɪk	170. workroom	wʌkwʊm	206. away	we~
137. sharp	ap	171. urinate	wiwɪ		weɪ
138. shirt	dʌt	172. yellow	lɛlʊ	207. elbow	ɛbu
139. shoe	du	173. yes	dɛt	208. empty	ɛbi
140. shopping	wɔbɪn	174. ladder	dɛdə	209. escape	gep
141. shoulder	dudə	175. lady	deɪdi	210. eye	aɪ
142. there	dɛ	176. ladybird	deɪdibət	211. on	ɔn
143. zebra	wibə	177. lash	dæt	212. open	ʊbu
144. chair	dɛ	178. later	dedə	213. other	ʌdə
145. chocolate	gɔgi~	179. lawnmower	mɔmə	214. out	aʊt
	gɔki	180. lazy	deɪdi	215. outside	aʊtdaɪt
146. church	dʌt	181. leg	gɛk	216. up	ʌp
147. jam	dɛm	182. Lego	gɛgu	217. uncle	ʌgʊ
148. John	dɔn	183. letter	dɛdə		

APPENDIX B–4

Jake

BACKGROUND: Jake is 2 years, 0 months of age and speaks a variety of midwestern English (Bleile, 1987).

WORD LIST

Intended Words	Jake	Intended Words	Jake
1. puppy	pʌpi	42. clown	kaʊn
2. pink	piŋk	43. book	bʊk
3. purple	pʊpʊ	44. ball	bɔ
4. picture	pɪtʃə	45. balls	bɔz
5. pig	p̊ɪg	46. bounce	baʊns
6. picnic table	pɪnɪteɪbʊ	47. bubbles	bʌbəs
7. please	pwiz	48. birthday	bʊfdeɪ
8. plate	pweɪt	49. birthday cake	bʊfdeɪkeɪk
9. teddy bear	tɛdi bɛ	50. boots	bus
10. teddy (bear)	tɛdi	51. baby	beɪbi
11. tail	teɪ.ə	52. Buster (a toy)	bʌstə
12. tear	tir	53. button	bʌʔn
13. turtle	tɝɾʊ	54. bunny	bʌni
14. toes	toʊz	55. bush	bʊs
15. two	tu	56. bugs	bʌgs
16. toothpaste	tupeɪs	57. bears	bɛz
17. triangle	twaɪ.æŋgʊ	58. back (n)	bæk
18. tree	twi	59. bye-bye	baɪ baɪ
19. tractor	twækʊ	60. bird	bʊd
20. trike	twaɪk	61. birds	bʊdz
21. twelve	twɛv	62. bicycle	baɪsɪkʊ
22. kitty	kɪɾi	63. box	baks
23. cat	kæt	64. board	bɔd
24. Cooly (a fish)	koʊwi	65. bananas	bænəs
25. carrot	kɛwɪt	66. Bert	bʊt
26. Katie	keɪɾi	67. break	bweɪk
27. cookie	kʊki	68. brown	bwaʊn
28. cookies	kʊkis	69. blue	bu
29. Curious George	kɪwi.əsdʒɔ	70. blueberry	bubɛwi
30. cows	kaʊz	71. black	bwæk
31. cards	kɑz	72. blackbirds	bwæk bʊz
32. Ken	kɛn	73. duck	dʌk
33. kangaroo	kæŋgəwu	74. daddy	dædi
34. kangaroos	kændəwus	75. daddy's	dædiz
35. cup	kʌp	76. Doc	dɑk
36. Cristopher	kwɪstəfʊ	77. don't	doʊn
37. cry	kwaɪ	78. dark	dɑk
38. cross (n)	kwɔs	79. Do Jo (a fish)	dʒoʊ dʒoʊ
39. crab (n)	kwæb	80. dandelion	dændiwaɪ.ɪn
40. close	kwoʊz	81. drink	dwiŋk
41. closet	kwɑzɪʔ	82. drive	dwaɪv

(continued)

WORD LIST (continued)

Intended Words	Jake	Intended Words	Jake
83. goat	goʊt	130. seals	si.əz
84. gopher	goʊfʊ	131. sea	si
85. green	gwin	132. circle	sɛˆkʊ
86. grandpa	gwæmpə	133. sleeping	sipi
87. grapes	gweɪps	134. slept	swɛpt
88. grass	gwæs	135. swing (v)	swiŋ
89. moon	mun	136. swimming	swɪmɪn
90. man	mæn	137. sweater	tɛwə
91. milk	mɛk	139. spoon	spun
92. monkey	mʌŋki	140. star	stɑ
93. monkeys	mʌŋkiz	141. stars	stɑds
94. motorcycle	moʊɾəsaɪkʊ	142. sticker	stɪkʊ
95. music	myuzɪk	143. stuck	stʌk
96. Mr. Kennedy's	mɪsəkɛniz	144. steps	stɛps
97. mommy's	mɑmiz	145. string	stwiŋ
98. move	muv	146. strawberries	stwɔbɛwiz
99. messy	mɛsi	147. stretch	stwɛ
100. Mickey Mouse	mɪki maʊs	148. square	skwɛ
101. Michael	maɪkʊ	149. smile	smaɪ.ə
102. Nancy	nætsi	150. smash	smæs
103. Neons (fish)	niɑ.nz	151. snap (v)	snæp
104. neat	nit	152. snowman	snoʊmæn
105. nose	noʊz	153. shout	saʊt
106. newts	nuts	154. shovel	ʃʌvʊ
107. no	noʊ	155. shampoo	ʃæmpu
108. nah ([næ])	næ	156. that	dæt
109. football	fɔbɔ	157. these	diz
110. fit	fɪt	158. there	dɛ
111. five	faɪv	159. zoo keeper	zu kipə
112. full	fʊ	160. chicken	tʃɪkɪn
113. fish	fɛs	161. Jake	dʒeɪk
114. fine	faɪn	162. Jake's	dʒeɪks
115. fast	fæ	163. juice	dʒus
116. face	feɪs	164. Jazzie (a cat)	dʒæzi
117. food	fud	165. Jazz(ie)	dʒæz
118. front	fwʌnt	166. hot	hɑt
119. frog	fwɔg	167. house	haʊs
120. friends	fwɛnz	168. Horse Face	hɔs feɪs
121. flower	faʊwə	169. hoop	hup
122. thank-you	sæŋku	170. heavy	hɛvi
123. three	fwi	171. Herky	hɛˆki
124. sour	saʊwə	172. hand	hæn
125. sit	sɪt	173. hands	hænz
126. set	sɛt	174. here	hɛ.ə
127. sunglasses	sʌngwæsɪz	175. hay	heɪ
128. circus	sɛˆkəs	176. him	hɪm
129. seal	siə	177. hungry	hʌŋgwi

(continued)

Intended Words	Jake	Intended Words	Jake
178. hi	haɪ	201. lion	waɪ.ɪn
179. white	waɪt	202. lotion	woʊsɪn
180. water	wɑɾə	203. loose	wus
181. walrus	wɔwəs	204. apple	æpʊ
182. whistle	wɪsʊ	205. orange (juice)	ɔɪns
183. watch (n)	wɑts	206. off	ɔf
184. one	wʌn	207. up	ʌp
185. woop	wʊp	208. elephant	ɛ.əfɛnt
186. woops	wʊps	209. elephants	ɛ.əfɪns
187. writing	waɪɾɪn	210. ok	oʊkeɪ
188. yellow	jɛdʊ	211. open	oʊpɪn
189. huge	jus	212. ice	aɪs
190. yes	jɛs	213. Ed	ɛd
191. yeah ([jeɪ])	jɔɪ	214. elbow	ɛboʊ
192. yah ([jæ])	jæ	215. (a)fraid	fweɪd
193. yep ([jɛp])	jɛp	216. accident	ækɪdɪn
194. red	wɛd	217. albums	æbəms
195. room	wum	218. excuse me	skuz mi
196. ready	wɛdi	219. orange	ɔɪns
197. rock	wɑk	220. umbrella	əmbwɛdə
198. rocks	wɑks	221. oval	oʊvʊ
199. ribbon	wɪbɪn	222. all gone	ɔ gɑn
200. light (n)	waɪt		

APPENDIX B–5

Tony

BACKGROUND: Tony is 3 years, 6 months of age, and is a native speaker of English who lives in Hawaii (Izuka, 1995).

WORD LIST

Intended Words	Tony	Intended Words	Tony
1. patch	✓	13. cup	✓
2. pig	✓	14. kangaroo	✓
3. pool	✓	15. ketchup	✓
4. prize	✓	16. cold	✓
5. cat	✓	17. crab	✓
6. car	✓	18. crayon	✓
7. cage	✓	19. clown	✓
8. cake	✓	20. clock	✓
9. candy	✓	21. ball	bɔ
10. carrot	✓	22. balloon	✓
11. coat	✓	23. bat	✓
12. cow	✓	24. bench	✓

(continued)

WORD LIST *(continued)*

Intended Words	Tony	Intended Words	Tony
25. bed	bɛ	71. square	✓
26. bird	✓	72. snake	✓
27. book	✓	73. sled	✓
28. bus	✓	74. slippers	✓
29. butterfly	✓	75. shower	✓
30. bugs	✓	76. shell	✓
31. boat	✓	77. sheep	✓
32. baby	✓	78. shoe	✓
33. berry	✓	79. van	✓
34. bathtub	bætəb	80. vest	✓
35. bridge	✓	81. the	✓
36. bread	✓	82. that	dæt
37. dinosaur	✓	83. zebra	✓
38. dish	✓	84. zipper	✓
39. dog	✓	85. zoo	✓
40. duck	✓	86. chair	✓
41. drum	✓	87. church	✓
42. guitar	✓	88. choo choo	tʃu tʃu
43. gun	✓	train	tʃreɪn
44. gate	✓	89. jelly	✓
45. goat	✓	90. judge	✓
46. grapes	✓	jacket	✓
47. meow	✓	91. giraffe	✓
48. milk	✓	92. hat	✓
49. mother	✓	93. hand	hæn
50. mouth	✓	94. hammer	✓
51. moose	✓	95. yard	✓
52. mat	✓	96. yellow	lɛloʊ
53. monkey	mʌnki	97. wagon	✓
54. nose	✓	98. watch	✓
55. knife	✓	99. witch	✓
56. fire	✓	100. radio	✓ ~
57. fork	✓		weɪdioʊ~
58. fish	✓		bweɪdioʊ
59. feather	✓	101. rain	✓
60. french fries	✓	102. reindeer	✓
61. flower	✓	103. rope	✓
62. thumb	tʌm	104. lamp	✓
63. sand	✓	105. leaf	✓
64. Santa Claus	sæntə klaʊs	106. light	✓
65. seal	✓	107. lion	✓
66. sun	✓	108. umbrella	✓
67. sandwich	sænwitʃ	109. elephant	✓
68. sticker	✓	110. arrow	ɑroʊ
69. star	✓	111. egg	✓
70. stove	✓	112. ankle	aɪnkl

APPENDIX B–6

Rikki

BACKGROUND: Rikki is 3 years, 6 months of age and is a native speaker of English who lives in Hawaii (Izuka, 1995).

WORD LIST

Intended Words	Rikki	Intended Words	Rikki
1. patch	✓	42. bridge	bwidʒ
2. pig	✓	43. broom	bwum
3. peanut butter	pinɔ bʌɾə	44. dish	✓
4. potatoes	✓	45. dive	✓
5. present	pwɛzɛnt	46. dog	✓
6. tail	tɛl	47. drum	dʒwʌm
7. teacher	titʃə	48. guitar	gɪtɑ
8. teeth	✓	49. gun	✓
9. telephone	✓	50. goat	✓
10. toes	✓	51. grass	✓
11. telescope	✓	52. glass	✓ ~
12. tub	✓		gəlæs
13. cap	✓	53. mouse	✓
14. kitty cat	✓	54. mother	mɑðə
15. cage	✓	55. mouth	✓
16. cake	✓	56. nose	✓
17. candy	✓	57. knife	✓
18. carrot	kæwɪt	58. fire	faɪ.ə
19. coat	✓	59. fork	foʊk
20. cow	✓	60. family	✓
21. cup	kɑp	61. feather	✓
22. campfire	✓	62. foot	fɑt
23. ketchup	✓	63. fish	fɛʃ
24. kite	✓	64. french fries	fwɛntʃ fwaɪz
25. key	✓	65. frog	fwɑg
26. crab	kwæb	66. flag	fwæg
27. crayon	kwæn	67. thumb	sʌm
28. clown	kwaʊn	68. sun	✓
29. clock	kəlɑk	69. Santa Claus	✓
30. ball	bɔ	70. seal	✓
31. balloon	bəwun	71. sink	✓
32. bat	✓	72. sandwich	sænwɪtʃ
33. bed	✓	73. spaghetti	spɑgɛɾi
34. boat	✓	74. spider	spaɪdʊ
35. bug	✓	75. star	stɑ
36. bathtub	✓	76. stove	✓
37. bathing suit	beɪɾɪŋ sut	77. stop sign	✓
38. baby bird	beɪbi bʊd	78. strawberry	ʃtrɔbɛwi
39. book	✓	79. string	ʃtrɪŋ
40. bus	✓	80. snake	✓
41. butterfly	✓	81. swimming pool	✓

(continued)

WORD LIST *(continued)*

Intended Words	Rikki	Intended Words	Rikki
82. sled	✓	101. house	✓
83. shampoo	✓	102. yard	dɔd
84. sheep	✓	103. yellow	lɛloʊ
85. shoe	✓	104. yawning	dɔnɪn
86. vest	vɛs	105. wagon	wægɪn
87. zebra	zibr̥ɑ~	106. witch	wɪtʃ
	zibwɑ	107. radio	weɪdi.oʊ
88. zero	ziwoʊ	108. rose	woʊs
89. zoo	✓	109. rain	weɪn
90. choo choo	tʃu tʃu	110. rocket ship	wɑkɪn ʃɪp
train	tʃweɪn	111. rope	woʊp
91. church	tʃʊtʃ	112. lamp	✓
92. jacket	✓	113. lemon	✓
93. jelly	✓	114. letter	lɛɾɪ
94. judge	✓	115. lion	laɪn
95. jump rope	dʒʌmp woʊp	116. lettuce	✓
96. giraffe	dʒɪwæf~	117. leaf	✓
	dʒəwæf	118. lunch	✓
96. hand	✓	119. little girl	wɪɾi gʊ
97. hat	✓	120. umbrella	✓
98. hop scotch	✓	121. oink	✓
99. hammer	hæmʊ	122. elephant	✓
100. hamburger	hæmbʊgʊ		

APPENDIX B–7

Diane

BACKGROUND: Diane is 3 years, 6 months of age, and is a native speaker of English who lives in Hawaii (Izuka, 1995).

WORD LIST

Intended Words	Diane	Intended Words	Diane	Intended Words	Diane
1. pocket	✓	13. train	tʃreɪn	25. clown	✓
2. pig	✓	14. kitten	✓	26. ball	✓
3. potato	✓	15. cage	✓	27. balloon	✓
4. tail	✓	16. cake	✓	28. bat	✓
5. teacher	✓	17. carrot	✓	29. bed	✓
6. tank top	✓	18. candy	✓	30. boat	✓
7. toes	✓	19. cow	✓	31. boy	✓
8. tomatoes	✓	20. kangaroo	✓	32. bicycle	✓
9. tire	✓	21. cup	✓	33. baby	✓
10. tub	✓	22. key	✓	34. books	✓
11. teeth	tit	23. kite	✓	35. bus	bʊs
12. telescope	✓	24. crab	✓	36. bathtub	bætəb

WORD LIST

Intended Words	Diane	Intended Words	Diane	Intended Words	Diane
37. bench	✓	67. thumb	tʌm	97. judge	✓
38. butterfly	✓	68. Santa Claus	✓	98. jump rope	✓
39. bridge	✓	69. seal	✓	99. giraffe	✓
40. dinosaur	✓	70. sun	✓	100. hand	✓
41. dish	✓	71. surprise	✓	101. hat	✓
42. dog	✓	72. sock	✓	102. hop scotch	hɑ ʃkwɑtʃ
43. drums	✓	73. sunflower	✓	103. yellow	lɛloʊ
44. gun	✓	74. spider	spaɪdʊ	104. yoyo	✓
45. gate	✓	75. star	✓	105. watch	✓
46. goat	✓	76. stove	stoʊf	106. witch	✓
47. grapes	✓	77. stop sign	✓	107. wagon	✓
48. grass	✓	78. string	ʃtriŋ	108. whale	✓
49. meow	✓	79. skirt	✓	109. world	✓
50. match	✓	80. snake	✓	110. water	✓
51. mouse	✓	81. swimming pool	✓	111. rabbit	✓
52. milk	✓	82. sled	✓	112. radio	✓
53. mother	mʌɾɚ	83. slide	✓	113. rain	✓
54. mouth	maʊt	84. slippers	slɪpʊ	114. rose	✓
55. noodles	✓	85. shampoo	✓	115. rope	✓
56. nose	✓	86. sheep	✓	116. lamp	✓
57. nail	nɛl	87. shoe	✓	117. leaf	✓
58. knife	✓	88. van	✓	118. lion	✓
59. fish	✓	89. vest	vɛs	119. lemonade	✓
60. five	✓	90. the mouse	də maʊs	120. leg	✓
61. fork	✓	91. zipper	✓	121. ladder	✓
62. feet	✓	92. zoo	✓	122. light	✓
63. feather	✓	93. chair	✓	123. umbrella	✓
64. flying saucer	✓	94. church	✓	124. elephant	✓
65. flag	✓	95. jelly	✓	125. ukulele	✓
66. flower	✓	96. jacket	✓		

APPENDIX B–8

Taylor

BACKGROUND: Taylor is 3 years, 6 months of age, and is a native speaker of English who lives in Hawaii (Izuka, 1995).

WORD LIST

Intended Words	Taylor	Intended Words	Taylor	Intended Words	Taylor
1. pants	✓	6. toes	toʊs	11. train	tʃreɪn
2. pen	✓	7. towel	taʊ	12. cat	✓
3. potato	✓	8. telescope	✓	13. car	✓
4. pool	pu	9. teeth	tiʔ	14. cowboy hat	✓
5. prison	✓	10. tub	tʌ	15. cake	✓

(continued)

WORD LIST (continued)

Intended Words	Taylor	Intended Words	Taylor	Intended Words	Taylor
16. carrot	kɛɾɪt~	54. guitar	✓	95. square	✓
	kʌwɪt	55. gun	✓	96. snake	✓
17. kangaroo	kɑŋgəwu	56. gate	✓	97. swing	✓
18. cup	✓	57. golf	✓	98. sled	✓
19. cow	✓	58. grapes	gweɪps	99. shirt	✓
20. coat	✓	59. grass	grɑs	100. sheep	✓
21. kitchen	✓	60. meow	✓	101. shoe	✓
22. cave	✓	61. moon	✓	102. van	✓
23. camera	✓	62. moose	✓	103. vest	vɪst
24. cookie	✓	63. milk	✓	104. the	dʌ
25. king	✓	64. mother	mʌɾə	105. zebra	ziwə
26. kite	✓	65. mouth	maʊ	106. zipper	✓
27. crab	kræb	66. noodles	nudls	107. zoo	✓
28. crayon	kweɪ.ən	67. nose	noʊs	108. chair	✓
29. clown	✓	68. knife	✓	109. church	✓
30. clothes	kloʊs~	69. fire	✓	110. children	✓
	kəloʊs	70. food	✓	111. jelly	✓
31. ball	bɔ	71. five	✓	112. judge	✓
32. bowl	boʊʔ	72. fork	✓	113. dragon	✓
33. boat	✓	73. feet	✓	114. hand	hæn
34. balloon	✓	74. feather	fɛɾɚ	115. house	✓
35. bat	✓	75. father	fɑɾɚ	116. yard	✓
36. bed	✓	76. finger	✓	117. yoyo	✓
37. belt	✓	77. fries	✓	118. yellow	lɛloʊ
38. bugs	✓	78. flower	✓	119. wagon	✓
39. button	✓	79. flag	✓	120. watch	✓
40. bottle	✓	80. thumb	tʌm	121. witch	✓
41. book	✓	81. thorn	✓	122. rabbit	✓
42. billy goat	✓	82. thing	✓	123. radio	✓
43. bus	✓	83. salad	sɑlɛd	124. ring	✓
44. butterfly	✓	84. sunshine	✓	125. rang	✓
45. bridge	brɛdʒ~	85. Santa Claus	sæntə klaʊ	126. rope	roʊp
	blɛdʒ	86. seal	✓	127. lamp	✓
46. broom	brʊm	87. sandwich	sænwɪtʃ	128. leaf	✓
47. dinosaur	✓	88. soap	✓	129. lady	✓
48. dish	dɪs	89. spider	spaɪdʊ	130. lion	✓
49. dive	daɪf	90. space	✓	131. letters	✓
50. dog	✓	91. star	✓	132. light	✓
51. duck	✓	92. stove	✓	133. umbrella	əmbwɛlə
52. drum	✓	93. steak fries	✓	134. eel	✓
53. dress	✓	94. steps	✓	135. elephant	✓

APPENDIX B–9

Ryan

BACKGROUND: Ryan is 5 years, 0 months of age, and a native speaker of English who lives in Hawaii (Izuka, 1995).

WORD LIST

Intended Words	Ryan	Intended Words	Ryan
1. person	✓	42. bird	✓
2. pig	✓	43. boat	✓
3. pocket	✓	44. book	✓
4. potato	✓	45. bottle	bɔɹl̩
5. pray	✓	46. butterfly	✓
6. presents	prɛsɛnts	47. bridge	✓
7. plate	✓	48. broom	✓
8. playground	✓	49. dinosaur	✓
9. please	✓	50. dish	✓
10. tail	✓	51. dive	daɪf
11. teacher	✓	52. dog	✓
12. teeth	✓	53. duck	✓
13. telephone	✓	54. dress	dʒirɛs
14. telescope	✓	55. drum	✓
15. toes	✓	56. gate	✓
16. cage	✓	57. guitar	✓
17. cake	✓	58. gun	✓
18. can	✓	59. goat	✓
19. candy	✓	60. grape	✓
20. car	✓	61. grass	✓
21. carrot	✓	62. meow	✓
22. cat	✓	63. microwave	✓
23. coat	✓	64. mother	✓
24. cockroach	✓	65. mouse	✓
25. cookie	✓	66. mouth	✓
26. cow	✓	67. nose	✓
27. cup	✓	68. knife	✓
28. kangaroo	✓	69. family	✓
29. ketchup	✓	70. feather	✓
30. king	✓	71. fire	✓
31. kite	✓	72. fish	✓
32. crayon	✓	73. fork	✓
33. clown	✓ ~ klin	74. french fries	✓
		75. frog	✓
34. baby	✓	76. flag	✓
35. ball	✓	77. flower	✓
36. balloon	✓	78. flying saucer	flaɪn saʊsə˞
37. bat	✓	79. thanksgiving	θæŋksgɪvɪn
38. bathtub	✓	80. thief	✓
39. bed	✓	81. thorn	✓
40. bicycle	✓	82. thermometer	✓
41. big	✓	83. thirsty	✓

(continued)

WORD LIST *(continued)*

Intended Words	Ryan	Intended Words	Ryan
84. thumb	sʌm~	130. that	✓
	✓	131. the	✓
85. Thursday	✓	132. them	✓
86. throw	✓	133. there	✓
87. safety pin	✓	134. this	✓
88. salt shaker	✓	135. those	✓
89. sandwich	sænwitʃ	136. Zack	✓
90. Santa Claus	sæntə kwɔz	137. zebra	✓
91. seal	✓	138. zero	✓
92. scissors	✓	139. zipper	✓
93. sign	✓	140. (the) zoo	zɑ zu~
94. six	sɛks		✓
95. sock	✓	141. xylophone	✓
96. soap	✓	142. chair	✓
97. circle	✓	143. cheese	✓
98. space	✓	144. church	✓
99. space shuttle	✓	145. choo choo	tʃu tʃu
100. spider	✓	train	tʃreɪn
101. splash	✓	146. judge	✓
102. splendid	✓	147. jump rope	✓
103. spray	✓	148. hand	hæn
104. spread	✓	149. hop scotch	✓
105. spring	✓	150. horse	✓
106. star	✓	151. yard	✓
107. stove	stoʊf	152. yellow	✓
108. strap	ʃtræp	153. yoyo	✓
109. straw	ʃtrɔ	154. watch	✓
110. stretch	ʃtrɛtʃ	155. witch	✓
111. school bus	✓	156. rabbit	✓
112. sky	✓	157. radio	✓
113. square	✓	158. rain	✓
114. squirrel	✓	159. raincoat	✓
115. snake	✓	160. rope	✓
116. swimming pool	✓	161. ribbon	✓
117. sled	✓	162. rose	✓
118. slide	✓	163. rug	✓
119. sharp	✓	164. lamp	✓
120. sheep	✓	165. lemon	✓
121. shell	✓	166. letter	✓
122. shirt	✓	167. light	✓
123. shoe	✓	168. leaf	✓
124. valentine	paʊlɛntaɪn	169. lion	✓
125. van	✓	170. little girl	✓
126. vest	✓	171. elephant	✓
127. vine	✓	172. ice skate	✓
128. violin	✓	173. one	✓
129. vitamin	✓	174. umbrella	✓

APPENDIX B–10

Max

BACKGROUND: Max is 5 years, 0 months of age, and a native speaker of English who lives in Hawaii (Izuka, 1995).

WORD LIST

Intended Words	Max	Intended Words	Max	Intended Words	Max
1. patch	pæts̬	42. book	✓	82. five	✓
2. pencil	pɛns̬ɪl	43. bugs	bʌgz	83. fork	✓ ~
3. pig	✓	44. bus	bʌs̬		✓
4. potatoes	pəteɪɾoʊz̬	45. butterfly	✓	84. french	fr̬ɛntʃ
5. pray	pr̬eɪ	46. bridge	bwɪdʒ	fries	fr̬aɪz
6. present	pr̬ɛz̬ɛnt	47. branch	✓	85. flag	✓
7. play	✓	48. broom	bwum~	86. flower	✓
8. please	✓ ~		✓	87. thorn	tʊrn
	plis	49. bright	✓	88. thumb	tʌm
9. teeth	tit	50. bloom	✓	89. throw	tʃr̬oʊ
10. tub	✓	51. blow	✓	90. three	tʃr̬i
11. tail	✓	52. dinosaur	daɪnəs̬ɔr	91. thread	tr̬ɛd
12. toe	✓	53. dish	dɪs̬	92. sun	s̬ʌn~
13. telescope	tɛlək°oʊp	54. dog	✓		sfʌn
14. twice	✓	55. duck	✓	93. sandwich	s̬ɑnwitʃ
15. truck	tʃr̬ʌk	56. drum	dr̬ʌm	94. Santa Claus	s̬æntə klɔz̬
16. train	tʃr̬eɪn	57. dress	dr̬ɛs̬	95. seal	s̬il
17. treat	tʃr̬it	58. drop	dr̬ɑp	96. soup	s̬up~
18. cage	✓	59. gate	geɪt		ʃup
19. cake	✓	60. gun	✓	97. space ship	p°eɪʃɪp
20. candy	✓	61. girl	gʊl~	98. space	p°eɪs
21. carrot	kær̬ɪt		✓	99. spaghetti	pɑgɛɾi
22. cat	✓	62. guitar	✓	100. spider	p°ʌɾɚ
23. coat	✓	63. goat	✓	101. splash	plɛʃ
24. cow	✓	64. grapes	✓	102. splendid	plɛndɪd
25. cup	✓	65. green	gr̬ɪn	103. spray	pr̬eɪ
26. kangaroo	kæŋgəwu	66. grass	gr̬æs̬	104. spread	pr̬ɛd
27. ketchup	✓	67. me	✓	105. splurge	plɝdʒ
28. queen	✓	68. matches	mætʃɛs̬	106. sprinkle	pr̬ɪŋkl̩
29. quick	✓	69. meow	✓	107. sky	k°aɪ
30. crow	kr̬oʊ	70. mouth	maʊt	108. square	kweɪr~
31. cream	kr̬im	71. milk	✓		gwɛr
32. crab	kr̬æb	72. mother	mʌɾʊ	109. squirrel	twɝl~
33. crayon	kr̬eɪjən	73. nail	✓		kwɝl
34. crutch	kr̬ʌtʃ	74. nose	noʊs̬	110. skate	k°eɪt
35. clown	✓	75. knife	✓	111. skunk	gʌŋk
36. balloon	✓	76. family	✓	112. skip	kɪp
37. bat	✓	77. feather	fɛtʊ	113. scream	kwim
38. bathing suit	beɪtɪŋ s̬ut	78. feet	✓	114. scratch	kr̬ætʃ
39. bathtub	bæɾəb	79. fire	✓	115. squirt	kwɝt
40. bed	bɛd̬	80. fish	fɪs̬	116. scrap	kr̬æp
41. boat	✓	81. face	feɪs̬	117. star	t°ɑr

(continued)

WORD LIST *(continued)*

Intended Words	Max	Intended Words	Max
118. stew	tu	152. zebra	zibwa
119. stop sign	tɑp s̺aɪn	153. zipper	zɪpʊ
120. stove	t°oʊv	154. zoo	✓
121. strap	tʃræp	155. chair	✓
122. straw	tr̥ɑ	156. chick	✓
123. stretch	ʃræp~	157. church	✓
	dr̥æp	158. judge	✓
124. street	tʃrit	159. jump rope	dʒʌmp r̥oʊp
125. smile	s̺maɪl	160. jeep	✓
126. smell	mɛl	161. hand	✓
127. snow	s̺noʊ	162. hat	✓
128. snake	s̺neɪk	163. hop scotch	hɑp kɑtʃ
129. swimming pool	s̺wɪmɪn pul~	164. house	haʊs
	fwɪmɪn pul	165. yard	jɑr̥d̥
130. sweater	s̺weɾʊ	166. yarn	✓
131. swim	fwɪm	167. yellow	✓
132. sweet	s̺wit	168. yoyo	✓
133. swamp	s̺wæmp	169. watch	✓
134. sled	s̺lɛd		wɑts̺
135. sleigh	s̺leɪ	170. witch	✓
136. slide	s̺laɪd	171. wagon	✓
137. slippers	s̺lɪpɚs̺	172. rabbit	ræbɪt̥
138. shell	s̺ɛl	173. radio	r̥eɪdi.oʊ
139. shoe	✓	174. red	r̥ɛd
140. sheep	s̺ip	175. rocks	r̥ɑks̺
141. shampoo	✓	176. rain	r̥eɪn
142. van	✓	177. rocket	r̥ɑkɛt
143. vase	veɪs̺	178. rope	r̥oʊp
144. vest	vɛs̺t̥	179. rose	r̥oʊs
145. voice	vɔɪs	180. lamp	✓
146. vine	✓	181. leaf	✓
147. vane	✓	182. lemon	✓
148. the	dʌ	183. lifesaver	laɪf s̺eɪvʊ
149. them	ðm̩	184. lion	laɪn
150. this	dɪs	185. umbrella	əmbr̥ɛlə
151. zap	zæp	186. elephant	✓

APPENDIX B–11

Shannon

BACKGROUND: Shannon is 5 years, 0 months of age, and a native speaker of English who lives in Hawaii (Izuka, 1995).

WORD LIST

Intended Words	Shannon	Intended Words	Shannon	Intended Words	Shannon
1. pants	✓	42. bus	✓	81. thumb	tʌm
2. patch	✓	43. butterfly	✓	82. thorn	toʊrn
3. pig	✓	44. bridge	✓	83. thin	tɪn
4. pink	✓	45. broom	✓	84. thread	tʃrɛd
5. potato	✓	46. dinosaur	✓	85. throw	tʃroʊ
6. pray	✓	47. dish	✓	86. sand	✓
7. present	✓	48. dive	daɪf	87. Santa Claus	✓
8. plate	✓	49. dog	✓	88. seal	✓
9. play	✓	50. duck	✓	89. soup	✓
10. tail	tɛl	51. drum	✓	90. sign	✓
11. teacher	✓		dʒrʌm	91. super	✓
12. teeth	tit	52. guitar	✓	92. space ship	✓
13. telescope	✓	53. gun	✓	93. space	✓
14. tub	✓	54. garage	✓	94. spaghetti	✓
15. train	tʃreɪn	55. gate	✓	95. spider	✓
16. tree	tʃri	56. giraffe	✓ ~	96. splendid	✓
17. cat	✓		dʒræf	97. splash	✓
18. cage	✓	57. girl	✓	98. spray	✓
19. cake	✓	58. goat	✓	99. spread	✓
20. candy	✓	59. grapes	✓	100. spring	✓
21. carrot	✓	60. grass	✓	101. sprinkle	✓
22. coat	✓	61. mail	✓	102. star	✓
23. cockroach	✓	62. meow	✓	103. stove	stoʊf
24. cookies	✓	63. milk	✓	104. strap	ʃtræp
25. cow	taʊ	64. mother	mʌɾɚ	105. string	ʃtrɪŋ-
26. cup	✓	65. mouth	maʊt		ʃtrɪŋ
27. kite	✓	66. nose	✓	106. skirt	✓
28. kangaroo	✓	67. numbers	✓	107. sky	✓
29. ketchup	✓	68. knife	✓	108. school bus	✓
30. coat	✓	69. fire	✓	109. square	skweɪr̥
31. queen	✓	70. feet	✓	110. squirrel	✓
32. crab	✓	71. fingers	✓	111. scratch	✓
33. crayon	✓	72. fork	✓	112. scream	✓
34. clown	✓	73. family	✓	113. snake	✓
35. ball	✓	74. feather	fɛɾʊ	114. swimming pool	✓
36. balloon	✓	75. face	✓	115. sled	✓
37. bat	✓	76. fish	✓	116. slide	✓
38. bed	✓	77. fruit	✓	117. slippers	slɪpɚs
39. bench	✓	78. french fries	✓	118. shampoo	✓
40. bird	✓	79. flag	✓	119. shark	✓
41. book	✓	80. flower	✓	120. sheep	✓

(continued)

WORD LIST *(continued)*

Intended Words	Shannon	Intended Words	Shannon
121. shirt	✓	145. yard	✓
122. shoes	ʃuz̥	146. yellow	✓
123. van	væn	147. wagon	✓
124. vase	✓	148. watch	✓
125. vest	✓	149. witch	✓
126. veto	✓	150. rabbit	✓
127. voice	✓	151. radio	✓
128. those	doʊz	152. rain	✓
129. the mouse	də maʊs	153. rock	✓
130. zebra	tsɪbrə	154. red	r̺ɛd
131. zipper	tsɪpɚ	155. river	✓
132. zoo	dʒu	156. rocket ship	✓
133. zap	✓	157. rope	r̺oʊp
134. chair	✓	158. lamp	✓
135. cheeseburger	✓	159. leaves	✓
136. church	✓	160. leaf	✓
137. jacket	✓	161. lemon	✓
138. jelly	✓	162. letter	✓
139. judge	dʒʌd̥ʒ	163. lighter	✓
140. jump	✓	164. lion	✓
141. hand	✓	165. umbrella	✓
142. hat	✓	166. elephant	✓
143. hop scotch	✓	167. oval	✓
144. house	✓		

APPENDIX B–12

Puuala

BACKGROUND: Puuala is 5 years, 0 months of age, and a native speaker of English who lives in Hawaii (Izuka, 1995).

WORD LIST

Intended Words	Puuala	Intended Words	Puuala	Intended Words	Puuala
1. patch	✓	13. tiger	✓	25. cage	✓
2. pig	✓	14. teacher	✓	26. candy	✓
3. potatoes	✓	15. teeth	tit	27. carrot	✓
4. pray	✓	16. train	tʃreɪn	28. coat	✓ ~
5. present	✓	17. truck	tʃrʌk		koʊd
6. president	✓	18. cat	✓	29. cockroach	✓
7. plate	✓	19. calendar	✓	30. cookies	✓
8. playground	✓	20. kangaroo	✓	31. cow	✓
9. play	✓	21. ketchup	✓	32. cowboy hat	✓
10. plug	✓	22. kid	✓	33. cup	✓
11. toes	toʊziz	23. kite	✓	34. queen	✓
12. tail	✓	24. kitten	✓	35. crab	✓

WORD LIST

Intended Words	Puuala	Intended Words	Puuala	Intended Words	Puuala
36. crayon	✓	83. fence	✓	129. sled	✓
37. clown	✓	84. fireplace	✓	130. slide	✓
38. ball	✓	85. fish	✓	131. slippers	✓
39. balloon	✓	86. fork	✓	132. shampoo	✓
40. bat	✓	87. flag	✓	133. sheep	✓
41. bathing suit	✓	88. flower	✓	134. shirt	✓
42. bathtub	✓	89. french fries	✓	135. valentine	✓
43. bed	✓	90. thanksgiving	✓	136. van	✓
44. bench	✓	91. thirty	✓	137. vase	✓
45. bird	✓	92. thermometer	✓	138. vest	✓
46. birthday cake	✓	93. thief	fif~	139. vine	✓
47. boat	✓		bif	140. violin	✓
48. body suit	✓	94. thirsty	✓	141. vitamin	✓
49. book	✓	95. thorns	✓	142. that	✓
50. Bugs Bunny	✓	96. thumb	✓	143. the mouse	✓
51. bunny rabbit	✓	97. Thursday	✓	144. the	✓
52. bus	✓	98. throw	✓	145. these	✓
53. butterfly	✓	99. safety pin	✓	146. them	✓
54. bridge	✓	100. salt shaker	✓	147. there	✓
55. broom	brʊm	101. sandwich	✓	148. those	✓
56. dinosaur	✓	102. Santa Claus	✓	149. zack	✓
57. dish	✓	103. scissors	✓	150. zip	✓
58. diving	✓	104. seagull	✓	151. zero	✓
59. dog	✓	105. seal	✓	152. zoo cage	✓
60. dog feet	✓	106. sock	✓	153. xylophone	✓
61. door	✓	107. soap	✓	154. chair	✓
62. duck	✓	108. space	✓	155. church	✓
63. drum	dʒrʌm	109. space ship	✓	156. giraffe	✓
64. gate	✓	110. spider	✓	157. jelly	✓
65. girl	✓	111. spray	✓	158. judge	✓
66. guitar	✓	112. spread	✓	159. jump rope	✓
67. gun	✓	113. splash	✓	160. hand	hæn
68. goat	✓	114. splendid	✓	161. hop scotch	✓
69. grapes	✓	115. star	✓	162. horse	✓
70. grass	✓	116. stop sign	✓	163. yard	✓
71. matches	✓	117. stove	✓	164. yawn	✓
72. meow	✓	118. strap	ʃtræp	165. yellow	✓
73. man	✓	119. straw	ʃtrɔ	166. yoyo	✓
74. mother	✓	120. string	ʃtrɪŋ	167. wagon	✓
75. mouse	✓	121. square	✓	168. watch	✓
76. mouth	✓	122. skirt	✓	169. wheels	✓
77. knife	✓	123. sky	✓	170. witch	✓
78. nail	✓	124. scratch	✓	171. radio	✓
79. nose	noʊs	125. scream	✓	172. rain coat	✓
80. noodles	✓	126. snake	✓	173. rain	✓
81. family	✓	127. snow	✓	174. rocket	✓
82. feather	✓	128. swimming pool	✓	175. rope	✓

(continued)

WORD LIST *(continued)*

Intended Words	Puuala	Intended Words	Puuala
176. ribbons	wɪbəns	181. letter	✓
177. rug	✓	182. light	✓
178. lamp	✓	183. lion	✓
179. leg	✓	184. umbrella	✓
180. lemon	✓	185. elephant	✓

APPENDIX
C

Longer Speech Samples From Clients With Articulation and Phonological Disorders

APPENDIX C–1

Dora

BACKGROUND: Dora is 2 years, 9 months of age (Wolfe, 1994). Dora's history is unremarkable except for having an older brother receiving services for speech prob- lems. Dora's hearing and language abilities are within normal limits.

WORD LIST

Intended Words	Dora	Intended Words	Dora	Intended Words	Dora
1. puppy	✓	7. carrot	tɛrət	13. bed	bɛ
2. pillow	piwoʊ	8. kitty cat	tɪʔi tæt	14. bananas	nænəz
3. pretty	pʌti	9. cup	tʌp	15. big	✓
4. telephone	bæbən	10. king	tɪn	16. bottle	bɑʔ
5. tricycle	taɪtɪtoʊ	11. cookie	tuti	17. Barney	✓
6. car	tɑr	12. bird	bʊd	18. bus	bʌʂ

(continued)

WORD LIST (continued)

Intended Words	Dora	Intended Words	Dora	Intended Words	Dora
19. ball	bɑ	34. scissors	tɪzɔz	49. hand	hæns
20. bib	bɪ	35. sun	tʌn	50. won	✓
21. blocks	bwɑʃ	36. soap	✓	51. was	✓
22. doggy	daʔi	37. socks	ʃɑʃ	52. what	wʌ
23. give	dɪb	38. stop	tɑp	53. window	✓
24. go	doʊ	39. sleeping	pipɪn	54. wagon	wædən
25. me	✓	40. shovel	ṣʌbḷ	55. light	waɪ
26. monster	mɑnsə	41. their	dɛr	56. leaf	wif
27. marker	mʌtɚs	42. that	dæt	57. low	woʊ
28. mine	✓	43. the	də	58. late	weɪt
29. no	✓	44. zoo	su	59. rain	reɪn
30. fishing	pɪʃɪn	45. zipper	ti	60. ride	waɪ
31. feathers	pɛʔəs	46. cheap	✓	61. ice cream	aɪtim
32. fits	bɪts	47. jungle	dʒʌnə	62. apple	æpu
33. find	faɪn	48. joke	dʒoʊt	63. egg	ɛd

APPENDIX C–2

Tess

BACKGROUND: Tess is 4 years, 4 months of age (Kim, 1995). Tess is bilingual (English and Korean) and is mildly delayed in the development of both languages. Tess's mother reports a normal prenatal and birth history, but that Tess did not say her first words until 2 years of age.

Tess is an only child and lives in an extended family household in which Korean is the primary language. Tess's exposure to English is primarily through her preschool. An audiological evaluation indicates hearing within normal limits.

WORD LIST

Intended Words	Tess	Intended Words	Tess	Intended Words	Tess
1. pineapple	paɪnæpʊ	13. cookie	tʊti	26. boat	bɔ
2. pink	pɪŋ	14. Cookie Monster	tuti mɑntə	27. boot	bu
3. play	peɪ	15. cow	taʊ	28. broken	bɔti.ɛn
4. popcorn	pɑtə	16. crab	dəwæb~	29. doctor	doʊktə
5. purple	pʌpʊ		tu. æ	30. dog	da
6. telephone	tɛpʊ	17. clown	taʊn	31. down	daʊ
7. turtle	tʌ	18. ball	bɑ	32. driving	daɪbɪŋ~
8. two	du~	19. banana	✓		daɪmɪŋ
	✓	20. bath	bæ	33. going	dɔ.ɪŋ
9. tree	təwi	21. bear	bɛ.ə	34. grandma	dænəma~
10. cannot	tænə	22. because	bita		dæma
11. cat	tæ~	23. bee	✓	35. McDonald's	mɪdanʊ
	tæt	24. big	bi		
12. coffee	tɑpi	25. bird	ba		

(continued)

WORD LIST *(continued)*

Intended Words	Tess	Intended Words	Tess	Intended Words	Tess
36. mommy	✓	50. sticker	tɪtə	64. wearing	wɛwi
37. morning	mɔni	51. strawberry	tɑbɛri	65. one	wã~
38. mouse	mɑʊ	52. skate	peɪt		wʌ
39. movie	mubi	53. chicken	tɪtɛm	66. rabbit	wæbɪ
40. no more	mɔmɔ.ə	54. Jihee [dʒíhi]	dihi	67. row	woʊ
41. fish	pɪti	55. juice	dyu	68. run away	wʌweɪ
42. five	paɪ	56. hair	hɛ.ə	69. lion	jaɪjɛ
43. flower	pɑʊwə	57. happy	hæpi	70. look	jut
44. four	pɔ.ə	58. have	hæb	71. apple	æpu
45. friend	pɛ̃	59. him	✓	72. eat	✓
46. three	twi	60. home	✓	73. eleven	ilɛbu
47. six	ti	61. homework	hɔmwõ	74. itchy	ɪti
48. sun	tʌ	62. washing	wɑtɪŋ	75. okay	oʊteɪ
49. star	tɑ	63. water	wɑtə	76. open	oʊp̃ɛ

APPENDIX C–3

Gavin

BACKGROUND: Gavin is 4 years, 8 months of age (Seo, 1995). At 14 months of age, Gavin was diagnosed with "failure to thrive." Gavin attends a special education program in a public preschool.

SPEECH SAMPLE

Words	Gavin	Words	Gavin	Words	Gavin	Words	Gavin
1. pig	bʌ~	13. bed	bʌ	25. santa	dʌ		
	pʌ	14. balloon	bʌ	26. soap	dʌ		
2. tiger	tʌ	15. dog	dʌ	27. spoon	pʌ		
3. truck	tʌ	16. door	bʌ~	28. shoes	bʌ		
4. tree	dʌ		dʌ	29. cheese	tʃʌ~		
5. carrot	bʌ~	17. girl	bʌ~		bʌ~		
	tæ		tʌ~		tʌ		
6. cat	tʌ~		dʌ	30. chair	bʌ~		
	tæ	18. green	bʌ		tʌ		
7. car	ʌ~	19. milk	bʌ	31. horse	hʌ		
	tʌ	20. monkey	mʌ	32. house	ʌ~		
8. cracker	tʌ	21. fish	bʌ~		hʌ		
9. boy	bʌ		fʌ	33. hat	dʌ		
10. baby	bʌ~	22. fork	bʌ	34. red	bʌ		
	bæ	23. fan	bʌ~	35. rabbit	wʌ~		
11. bird	bʌ		bæ		wæ		
12. boat	bʌ	24. sandwich	ʃæ				

APPENDIX C–4

Stacy

BACKGROUND: Stacy is 5 years, 2 months of age (Bleile, 1995). Stacy's medical, social, and developmental history are unremarkable. Results of a speech-language evalua- tion indicate that Stacy's only area of deficit is in articulation and phonological development.

WORD LIST

Intended Words	Stacy	Stimulability Testing	Intended Words	Stacy	Stimulability Testing
1. pipe	✓		39. nails	neɪs	
2. Power Rangers	paʊwʊweɪndəs		40. feather	fɛdʊz	
3. potatoes	✓		41. fork	✓	
4. pencil	pɛnsʊ		42. fish	fɪs	fɪʃ
5. toothbrush	tubwəs	tubwəʃ	43. flowers	flaʊwʊz	
6. teeth	tit		44. flag	fjæg	fjæg
7. toy kitty	✓		45. thumb	fʌm	fʌm
8. TV	✓		46. scissors	sɪzɪs	
9. table	teɪbʊ		47. sandwich	sæwɪs	
10. train	sweɪn	sweɪn	48. saw	✓	
11. can	✓		49. swing	fʊwɪŋ~	
12. keys	✓			fwɪŋ	
13. kitty	✓		50. spoon	pud	pud
14. cup	✓		51. stove	toʊv	toʊv
15. comb	✓		52. stars	tɔz	tɔz
16. cake	✓		53. skates	keɪs	
17. cat	kyæt	kæt	54. shoe	su	ʃu
18. car	kɑr		55. vacuum	væki.ə	
19. carrots	kæwɪs		56. zipper	✓	
20. crackers	kwækʊz	kwækʊz	57. chair	sɛr	sɛr
21. crayons	kwænz	kwænz	58. jars	zɑz	zɑz
22. clock	kjæk	kjæk	59. wagon	✓	
23. book	✓		60. house	✓	
24. baby	✓		61. hammer	hæmʊ	
25. (bath)tub	bætəb		62. hangers	hæŋgʊ	
26. bed	✓		63. hat	✓	
27. bananas	✓		64. witch	wɪs	wɪs
28. balloons	✓		65. whistle	wɪs	
29. bell	✓		66. lion	jaɪn	jaɪn
30. brush	bwʌs		67. ladder	jædʊ	
31. blocks	bjɑks	bjɑks	68. lamp	jæmp	jæmp
32. blue	bju		69. radio	weɪdi.oʊ	weɪdi.oʊ
33. dog	✓		70. red	wɛd	
34. gun	✓		71. elephant	✓	
35. green	gwin		72. orange	ɔɪns	
36. monkey	✓		73. angels	ænzʊs	
37. matches	mæsɪz	mæsɪz	74. egg	✓	
38. knife	✓		75. apple	æpʊ	

APPENDIX C–5

Cain

BACKGROUND: Cain is 5 years, 7 months of age (Kim, 1995). Cain's medical history is significant for seizures for which he receives medication (Phenobarbital). Cain is enrolled in a full-time, self-contained special education classroom where he receives speech and physical therapy services.

WORD LIST

Word	Cain	Word	Cain	Word	Cain
1. pajamas	dʒɑmɑs	30. gun	dʌn	59. small	h̃mɑ
2. pencils	pɛnhɔs	31. matches	✓	60. smoke	h̃moʊk
3. present	prɛh͂ɛn	32. milk	mɛ̃	61. snail	h̃neɪ.ə
4. telephone	tɛəhoʊn	33. monster	mãnhtɚ	62. snake	h̃neɪʔ~
5. tiger	taɪhɚ	34. knife	naɪh		h̃neɪk
6. toothbrush	tubrəʃ	35. fast	hæs	63. snow	h̃noʊ
7. touch	tʌʃ	36. feather	hɛdɚ	64. snowman	h̃noʊ mæn
8. car	tɑr	37. finger	hɪndɚ	65. sleep	hip
9. carrot	tɛrɪt	38. fire	hwaɪr	66. sleeping	hĩpiŋ
10. Kim	tɪm	39. fishing	hɪʃɪŋ	67. slow	hɔ
11. come	tʌm	40. five	haɪf	68. shovel	ʃʌbu
12. cool	hu.ə	41. four	hwɔr	69. vacuum	bæhyu
13. cup	hʌ~	42. flag	hwæ	70. this	dɪs
	hʌp	43. thumb	hʌm	71. zipper	hɪʔpɚ
14. cut	tʌt	44. Santa Claus	tænə twɔs	72. chickens	tʃɪʔɛns
15. Christmas tree	hmɪs hmɪs	45. scissors	hɪhɚs	73. church	✓
	tʃri	46. cereal	hɪwɪ.ɔ	74. jump	✓
16. cross	trɑs	47. see	h̃ĩ	75. house	hoʊʃ
17. bath	✓	48. sisters	hʌhɚs	76. yellow	jɛjoʊ
18. bathtub	bætəb	49. sit	hɪʔ	77. wagon	wæhɛn
19. bed	✓	50. surfing	hɚhɪŋ	78. wheel	wi.ʊ
20. bell	bɛ.ə	51. spaghetti	hʌtɛ.i~	79. window	wɛndoʊ
21. boat	✓		hɪtɛ.i	80. rabbit	✓
22. bother	bɑ.ɚ	52. spoon	bun	81. ring	✓
23. bracelet	breɪhjɛt	53. stars	dɑrs	82. lamp	jæm
24. brush	bʌʃ	54. stove	toʊv	83. light	jaɪt
25. blue	bwu	55. skating	teɪ.i	84. long	jɑn
26. duck	dʌ	56. skis	tis	85. airplane	ɛrpweɪn
27. drum	dʒrʌm	57. skunk	tʌŋk	86. orange	✓
28. go	doʊ	58. squirrel	twɚ.əl	87. over	oʊ.ɚ
29. got	dɑt				

APPENDIX C–6

Bobby

BACKGROUND: Bobby is 5 years, 7 months of age (Seo, 1995). Bobby attends a public elementary school, and wears bilateral PE tubes because of a history of chronic otitis media.

WORD LIST

Intended Words	Bobby	Intended Words	Bobby	Intended Words	Bobby
1. pair	✓	39. dolly	✓	77. soft	sɔf
2. pig	✓	40. dress	dʒwɛs	78. some	✓
3. pretty	pwɪɾi	41. dry	dʒwaɪ	79. sun	✓
4. play	pweɪ	42. get	dɛt	80. suprise	sɑpwaɪz
5. table	teɪboʊ	43. girl	✓	81. spill	pɪl
6. teeth	tit	44. give	dɪv	82. spray	pweɪ
7. T.V.	✓	45. go	doʊ	83. splash	pwæs
8. two	✓	46. going	doʊ.ɪŋ	84. stairs	teɪrz
9. twin	✓	47. gum	dʌm	85. stove	toʊv
10. trees	tʃwiz	48. gun	dʌn	86. strap	tʃwæp
11. cake	teɪk	49. green	gwin	87. straw	tʃwɔ
12. car	tɑr	50. grow	gwoʊ	88. sky	taɪ
13. carrots	tærɛts	51. glue	gwu	89. square	kweɪr
14. cat	tæt	52. mask	mæs	90. scream	kwim
15. cold	toʊd	53. me	✓	91. smell	✓
16. comb	toʊm	54. monkey	mʌnki	92. snail	✓
17. cornflake	toʊrnfweɪt	55. most	moʊs	93. swim	✓
18. country	tʌntʃwi	56. mouth	maʊt	94. swing	wɪŋ
19. cow	taʊ	57. mustard	✓	95. sleep	✓
20. cup	tʌp	58. knife	✓	96. shrimp	swɪmp
21. key	✓	59. nest	nɛs	97. that	dæt
22. king	tɪŋ	60. nicely	✓	98. the	dʌ
23. kiss	tɪs	61. nine	✓	99. zero	zɪwoʊ
24. Quick	✓	62. no	✓	100. zip	✓
25. cry	tʃwaɪ	63. nose	✓	101. chair	✓
26. clock	kwɑk	64. fish	fɪs	102. choo-choo	tʃu +ʃu
27. baby	✓	65. five	✓	train	tʃweɪn
28. ball	bɔ	66. fork	f	103. jump rope	dʒʌmp woʊp
29. basket	bæstɪt	67. four	✓	104. horse	✓
30. bathtub	✓	68. fruit	fwut	105. house	✓
31. between	✓	69. fly	fwaɪ	106. yam	✓
32. bike	✓	70. three	θwi	107. yeah	✓
33. bird	✓	71. thumb	tʌm	108. yellow	lɛloʊ
34. books	✓	72. Santa Claus	sæntə tɔs	109. yes	✓
35. brain	bweɪn	73. second	sɛkɛn	110. yo	✓
36. brush	bwʌs	74. secret	sikwɛt	111. yuck	✓
37. blow	bwoʊ	75. seven	✓	112. wagon	✓
38. dog	✓	76. six	✓	113. wasp	wɑs

(continued)

WORD LIST (continued)

Intended Words	Bobby	Intended Words	Bobby	Intended Words	Bobby
114. watch	wɑts	124. Robin	wɑbɪn	134. apply	əpweɪ
115. weekly	wiki	125. roll	woʊ	135. ear	i
116. wobbling	wɑbəlɪŋ	126. round	waʊn	136. eggs	✓
117. worms	✓	127. rust	wʌs	137. ice cream	aɪs kwim
118. whisper	✓	128. ladder	✓	138. iceman	✓
119. whistle	wɪsoʊ	129. last	læs	139. ugly	ʌgəli
120. raindrop	weɪndwɑp	130. laundry	lɑndʒri	140. umbrella	əmbwɛlə
121. red	wɛd	131. looking	✓	141. unsnap	✓
122. rich	wɪts	132. afraid	əfweɪd	142. upswing	✓
123. ring	wɪŋ	133. agree	✓		

APPENDIX C–7

Kelly

BACKGROUND: Kelly is 5 years, 10 months of age (Kim, 1995). Kelly's mother reports an unremarkable pregnancy and birth history, and hearing is within normal limits.

Kelly's preschool teacher reports that Kelly does well in school, but that her speech calls attention to itself.

WORD LIST

Word	Kelly	Word	Kelly	Word	Kelly
1. patch	✓	20. balloon	✓	39. mommy	✓
2. pig	✓	21. bat	✓	40. mouth	maʊt
3. potatoes	✓	22. bed	✓	41. knife	naɪp
4. teeth	tit	23. boat	✓	42. nose	noʊt~
5. telescope	tɛlɛkoʊp	24. book	✓		noʊd
6. tub	✓	25. boss	bɑts	43. feather	wɛdə
7. train	tʃreɪn	26. bus	bɑts	44. fire	waɪyə
8. cage	✓	27. butterfly	bʌdəwaɪ	45. fish	wɪt
9. cake	✓	28. bridge	bwɪdʒ	46. flag	wæg
10. candy	✓	29. dinosaur	daɪnətɔ	47. thumb	tʌm
11. kangaroo	kæŋgəwu	30. dish	dɪts	48. saw	tɑ
12. carrot	kɛwɛt	31. diving	daɪbɪŋ	49. Santa Claus	tæntə klɑd
13. cat	✓	32. dog	✓	50. seal	tiə
14. coat	✓	33. duck	✓	51. sun	tʌn
15. cow	✓	34. gate	✓	52. star	tɑ
16. cup	✓	35. goat	✓	53. stove	toʊb
17. crab	kwæb	36. gun	✓	54. snake	neɪk
18. crayon	kweɪ.ɑn	37. meow	✓	55. sled	tɛd
19. clown	✓	38. milk	mɪək	56. sheep	tip

(continued)

WORD LIST (continued)

Word	Kelly	Word	Kelly	Word	Kelly
57. shoe	tu	67. judge	✓	78. radio	✓
58. van	✓	68. hand	✓	79. rain	✓ ~
59. vest	vɛt	69. hat	hæt		weɪn
60. the	dɑ	70. horse	hɔrti	80. rope	woʊp
61. they	deɪ	71. house	haʊt	81. lamp	✓
62. zipper	dɪpə	72. yard	jɑd	82. leaf	lip
63. zoo	du	73. yellow	lɛloʊ	83. lion	✓
64. chair	tʃɛ.ə	74. wagon	✓	84. elephant	ɛləwɛnt
65. church	tʃʌtʃ	75. watch	✓	85. umbrella	əmbwɛlə
66. jelly	✓	76. wheel	wiə		
		77. rabbit	wæbɪt		

APPENDIX C–8

Billy

BACKGROUND: Billy is 6 years, 8 months of age (Wolfe, 1994). Billy's medical, developmental, and social history are unremarkable. Billy's hearing is within normal limits and he scores at the 94th percentile in receptive vocabulary on the Peabody Picture Vocabulary Test-Revised (Dunn & Dunn, 1981).

WORD LIST

Intended Words	Billy	Intended Words	Billy	Intended Words	Billy
1. pajamas	pədʒæməz	15. green	gwin	29. lamp	✓
2. pencils	pɪnsɪlz	16. great	grɛt	30. ring	rɪŋ
3. telephone	✓	17. fishing	✓	31. rabbit	ræbət
4. car	✓	18. finger	fɪŋɚ	32. house	✓
5. carrot	kɛrət	19. vacuum	✓	33. window	✓
6. cream	✓	20. thumb	✓	34. wagon	✓
7. cry	kwaɪ	21. this	✓	35. wheel	✓
8. bathtub	✓	22. stove	✓	36. yellow	✓
9. bath	✓	23. shovel	✓	37. airplane	ɛpleɪn
10. blue	✓	24. zipper	zɪpə	38. orange	ɔndʒ
11. brush	bʌʃ	25. jumping	✓	39. American	əmɛrəkn̩
12. duck	✓	26. chicken	✓	flag	flæg
13. drum	drʌm	27. knife	✓		
14. gun	✓	28. matches	✓		

PROBE WORDS

Intended Words	Billy	Intended Words	Billy	Intended Words	Billy
1. rain	✓	3. run	rʌn	5. story	✓
2. row	woʊ	4. root	✓	6. merry	✓

(continued)

PROBE WORDS (*continued*)

Intended Words	Billy	Intended Words	Billy	Intended Words	Billy
7. hero	✓	11. light	✓	15. ring	rɪŋ
8. car	✓	12. row	woʊ	16. low	✓
9. bear	✓	13. log	✓	17. ray	reɪ
10. air	✓	14. leaf	✓	18. late	✓

APPENDIX C–9

Dee

BACKGROUND: Dee is 7 years, 5 months of age (Lee, 1994). Dee was diagnosed with a communication disorder at 3 years of age. Dee receives speech-language services twice a week through a speech and hearing clinic.

WORD LIST

Intended Words	Dee	Intended Words	Dee	Intended Words	Dee
1. patch	✓	28. dinosaur	✓	55. shoe	✓
2. pig	✓	29. dish	✓	56. van	✓
3. potatoes	✓	30. dive	✓	57. vest	✓
4. teeth	tit	31. dog	✓	58. this	dɪs
5. telescope	tɛləkoʊp	32. duck	✓	59. the	də
6. tub	✓	33. gate	deɪt	60. zipper	zɪpə
7. train	tʃɛn	34. goat	✓	61. zoo	✓
8. cage	✓	35. gun	✓	62. chair	tʃɛ.ə
9. cake	keɪt	36. meow	miwaʊ	63. church	tʃɝ
10. candy	tændi	37. milk	✓	64. jelly	✓
11. kangaroo	tændəwə	38. mother	mʌdʊ	65. judge	dʒʌd
12. carrots	kæwəts	39. mouth	maʊt	66. hand	✓
13. cat	✓	40. knife	naɪ	67. hat	✓
14. cup	✓	41. nose	✓	68. yard	jʌd
15. coat	✓	42. feather	fɛdʊ	69. yellow	lɛloʊ
16. cow	✓	43. fish	✓	70. wagon	✓
17. crab	kæb	44. fire	faɪ.ə	71. watch	✓
18. crayon	kɛwən	45. flag	fæg	72. rabbit	wæbɪt
19. clown	kaʊn	46. thumb	tʌm	73. radio	weɪdi.oʊ
20. balloon	✓	47. Santa Claus	sæntə kɔz	74. rain	weɪn
21. bat	✓	48. seal	si.ə	75. rope	woʊp
22. bed	✓	49. sun	✓	76. lamp	✓
23. boat	✓	50. star	tɑ.ə	77. leaf	✓
24. book	✓	51. stove	toʊv	78. lion	✓
25. bus	✓	52. snake	neɪk	79. elephant	✓
26. butterfly	bʌdəfaɪ	53. sled	sɛd	80. umbrella	əmbwɛji.ə
27. bridge	bɪdʒ	54. sheep	✓		

APPENDIX
D

Transcription Conventions

TRANSCRIPTION CONVENTIONS

The transcriptions in this workbook generally follow the conventions of the International Phonetic Association. The following are conventions specific to this workbook.

1. **Syllable Boundaries**
   A. Syllable boundaries are those of the adult language except where noted. For example, the syllable boundary of *between* in the adult language comes between [i] and [t]. The syllable boundary would not be indicated if a client pronounces *between* with the same syllable boundary. A period is used to indicate syllable boundaries that differ from those in the adult language. For example, a pronunciation of *between* with the syllable boundary between [t] and [w] (a highly unlikely pronunciation) would be transcribed [bit.win].
   B. A period is used to indicate syllable boundaries when possibly ambiguous sequences of vowel symbols occur. For example, [iu] (for *me too*) might be either a diphthong or two syllables. If two syllables, it would be transcribed [i.u].

2. **Vowels**
   A. A sequence of two vowels in the same syllable should be interpreted as a diphthong. A vowel followed by a raised vowel in the same syllable should be interpreted as a vowel followed by a brief off-glide.
   B. A single vowel symbol indicates a pure vowel (monothong) and two vowel symbols in the same syllable indicate a diphthong. For example, if *bait* is transcribed [bet] for one client and [beɪt] for another, the vowel is a monothong for the first client and a diphthong for the second.

3. **Aspiration**
   A. Persons in Stage 2 are not expected to pronounce voiceless stops with English-like aspiration. Unless indicated by a raised "h," voiceless stops in the speech of persons in Stage 2 are pronounced without aspiration. For example, for persons in Stage 2 the consonant in [pu] for *Pooh* should be interpreted as being unaspirated.
   B. Persons in Stage 3 or 4 are expected to pronounce voiceless stops with English-like aspiration. For persons in these stages the consonant in [pu] for *Pooh* should be interpreted as aspirated.

Index

CPSIA information can be obtained
at www.ICGtesting.com
Printed in the USA
FFOW031106211112
334FF